My L   xic

DATE DUE

HAWORTH Titles of Related Interest

Anorexia Nervosa and Recovery: A Hunger for Meaning
by Karen Way

*The Bulimic College Student: Evaluation, Treatment,
and Prevention* edited by Leighton C. Whitaker and William
N. Davis

Fat Oppression and Psychotherapy: A Feminist Perspective
edited by Laura S. Brown and Esther D. Rothblum

Obesity and the Family edited by David J. Kallen
and Marvin B. Sussman

*Women's Conflicts about Eating and Sexuality: The
Relationship Between Food and Sex* by Rosalyn Meadow
and Lillie Weiss

The Evaluation and Treatment of Eating Disorders
edited by Diane Gibson

My Life
as a Male Anorexic

Michael Krasnow

Harrington Park Press
An Imprint of The Haworth Press, Inc.
New York • London

Published by

Harrington Park Press, an imprint of The Haworth Press, Inc., 10 Alice Street, Binghamton, NY
13904-1580

Library of Congress Cataloging-in-Publication Data

Krasnow, Michael.
   My life as a male anorexic / Michael Krasnow.
      p.   cm.
   ISBN 1-56023-883-6 (alk. paper)
    1. Krasnow, Michael. 2. Anorexia nervosa–Patients–Biography. I. Title.
RC552.A5K73   1996
616.85′262′0092–dc20
[B]   95-43399
                                                       CIP

In memory of my father

and

In honor of my mother

ABOUT THE AUTHOR

Michael Krasnow was born in Rochester, NY in 1969 and grew up in Framingham, MA. He has suffered from anorexia nervosa for more than ten years. He currently resides in Hollywood, FL.

CONTENTS

Preface

I will never forget the first time I saw Michael in 1988. I was asked to consult his psychiatrist, Dr. Stephen Wiener, concerning Michael's medical condition while Michael was a patient at Bournewood Hospital, a psychiatric hospital in the Boston area. On seeing Michael, I immediately thought of the grotesque images of concentration camp victims from World War II. Michael regarded me warily. He politely answered my medical questions, and allowed me to examine him. Although skeletal, and obviously emaciated, the remainder of his physical examination was normal. At age 18, he was already an experienced patient, having undergone several hospitalizations and treatment with several psychiatrists. He was 82 pounds, felt fat, and was insisting on his right to lose more weight. All attempts at rational discourse, as well as psychotherapy, had not broken through his obsessional desire to lose weight.

Subsequently, Michael underwent three tumultuous medical hospitalizations at Newton-Wellesley Hospital. The hospital discharge summaries (see Appendix II) illuminate the critical medical situation in which there is intense conflict between Michael's desire to control his weight and his physician's desperate determination to save his life. This resulted in a fierce medical battle, which ultimately resulted in a sort of truce, where Michael remained grossly underweight but agreed to regular medical monitoring in my office. The truce actually resulted in a new doctor-patient relationship based on respect and trust, and the understanding Michael had that I did care about his living and well-being. After these stormy hospitalizations, Michael appeared to stabilize at 74 1/2 pounds and was seen by me in my office at regular intervals with his mother at his side. He insisted on maintaining his low weight.

I believe that the positive relationship between Michael and his treaters, as acknowledged by Michael himself in his life story, in other words, the positive transference, has allowed him to go on living. He was able to achieve a physiological as well as a psychological "steady-state" compatible with life. Of course, it is on his own terms.

It appears to me that Michael's being in control of his anorexia as well as the anorexia itself has been the central achievement of his life. In that sense, the publication of this book both validates and nourishes him.

Theodore E. Spielberg, MD

Chapter 1

Introduction

For some time now, my mother has been encouraging me to write a book about my screwed-up life and my experiences with anorexia nervosa and depression. I've never given this idea much consideration. Because of the depression, I just haven't had the motivation. However, now that I'm not working, I figure I may as well give it a shot. After all, it's been around two years since I stopped working; most of this time has been spent sitting in a chair in my apartment, staring at the wall. Talk about a waste. These past couple of years epitomize my life–a total waste.

First, the facts that make me an "official" anorexic. The so-called professionals, your $100-per-hour, know-it-all doctors, will list many symptoms and characteristics of anorexia. The bottom line is that I am 5'9" and feel fat, despite weighing only 75 pounds. Just for the record, I am white, American, Jewish, and twenty-five years old. I live in Hollywood, Florida, and in case you weren't paying attention to the cover, my name is Michael Krasnow. What sets me aside from most other anorexics is that I am male.

For years, anorexia existed, but very few people knew of it. Women who suffered from it did not realize that they were not alone. Eventually, as more became known and anorexia became more publicized, a greater number of women came forward to seek help, no longer feeling that they would be considered strange or outcasts from society. Maybe with the publication of this book, more men with the problem will realize that they are not alone either, and that they do not suffer from a "woman's disease." They can come forward without worrying about embarrassment.

Who knows? Maybe as a result of this book, I'll end up on television. Perhaps you just saw me on a talk show, and that's why you're reading this book. The more publicity I can get, the better. Each book that is sold will make that many more people aware of the serious problem of male anorexia. And the more people that know, the more demand there will be to help those with this problem.

Almost all books and articles about anorexia deal with females. However, since this book is about a male anorexic, namely myself, I will use masculine pronouns throughout the story.

So much for preliminaries. It is time to tell you about myself. I guess the most logical way of doing this is to start at the beginning.

Chapter 2

Feeling Fat

I suppose I had a typical childhood. Born in Rochester, New York, on April 27, 1969, I moved to Framingham, Massachusetts, when I was two months old and lived there for about twenty-two years. I enjoyed being with my friends and family, loved to read and play sports, had a hobby (comic books) and a newspaper route, watched TV, idolized Larry Bird and the Boston Celtics, and had no worries. I was an all-around average child. My one unusual characteristic was that I felt fat from as early as age eleven, when I was in the sixth grade. I occasionally mentioned this feeling to my parents and grandparents, but not with any seriousness. I used to joke with them that I was going to diet. Understandably, no one paid any attention. After all, I was of average weight. Actually, I was less than average, the type of child that others refer to as "so skinny."

When I speak of feeling fat, what I mean is that when I look down at my stomach, I see it as sticking out or being bloated.

In 1980, my brother, Neil, got a summer job as an apprentice at the Cape Cod Melody Tent, a theatre in Hyannis, Massachusetts. My only sibling, Neil is about three and a half years older than I. Although we have grown closer over the years, Neil and I were never very close as children. No special reason, really. I guess we just had different tastes. Neil loved the theatre; I loved sports. Anyway, this would be the first of four consecutive summers that I spent at the Cape. I did not like the Cape and told my parents this, but I had no choice. Each summer, my parents and grandparents rented a cottage and dragged me down there with them.

It was during these summers that I started to wonder why I felt fat. I knew that statistically I wasn't fat, and everyone told me how skinny I was. I decided to try dieting, but never kept to it for more than a couple of days (I figured it was a lack of willpower). Because I never stuck to a diet, no one paid much attention.

At this time, my feelings of being fat began to affect my activities. Before, I had felt fat, but had not been influenced by these feelings. Now, I would not go to the beach because I did not want to take off my shirt. Without a shirt, I'd see my stomach and feel fat; I believed others who saw my stomach would also think I looked fat. When I could not make up an excuse for not going to the beach, I kept my shirt on, or if I had to take it off, I sucked in my gut and held it.

Sucking in my gut became a way of life. I played basketball in my temple's youth league. In practice, we scrimmaged as "shirts" and "skins." I hated being on the "skins" team. When I was, I was unable to focus on the game, being too preoccupied with thinking about sucking in my gut.

Two specific games that stand out in my mind are the championship games, which were shown on local cable television. During these games, worried about looking fat on TV, I reminded myself–suck in your gut.

Some more examples? How about June 1983, more specifically, my last day of the eighth grade and middle school. A friend invited me to a pool party. Yes, I enjoyed myself–had a great time. However, during the entire party, in the back of my mind, I was thinking, "Don't forget to suck in your gut."

Another occasion that I recall is my bar mitzvah. While standing on the bimah (a bimah in a temple is the equivalent of a pulpit in a church), with everyone watching me, I felt fat. Sure enough, I sucked in my gut.

At my bar mitzvah and other parties, I was reluctant to dance. I felt fat when someone's hands were around my waist. It made me embarrassed and ashamed to think that others were saying to themselves, "Hmm, he's fat–has a real big waist." I felt uneasy and self-conscious. When I did dance, it was usually with my mother, grandmothers, or other family.

I occasionally danced with a girl my age, but not too often. Not that I didn't want to, I just lacked confidence around girls— was too shy and too scared to ask. Because of the shyness, the fear, and the embarrassment caused by having someone's hands around my waist, I just decided not to dance.

Actually, feeling fat may not have had anything to do with my reluctance to dance. After all, I could have simply sucked in my gut. I don't think I would have danced even if I had felt skinny. I mean, I really, really wanted to. I was just too scared to ask, too scared that the girl would say no, and that I'd feel foolish. Are any of you girls who knew me at that age reading this? If so, what's going through your minds? Did you think I was "cool" or a loser? Or did you not care one way or the other? Would you have danced? I suppose I'm just curious. My guess, only a guess, is that you probably did not care one way or the other.

I have given you a few examples of my feeling fat. There are many more, but there's no reason to list each one. They all follow the same pattern, and I'm sure you get the general idea. However, I would like to tell of just one other situation.

My father was a member of a health club, Racquetball Five-O. I had a very close relationship with my father. He was the greatest man to ever walk the face of this earth, and I'll tell you more about him in a little while. Anyway, I went to this health club with my dad once or twice a week. When I was in the locker room, naked, I always sucked in my gut.

I am singling out these locker-room occasions because they lead to an interesting observation. Standing in that locker room, I saw the other men around me as being fat. In other words, I felt fat, but my disillusionment was not limited to myself. Most anorexics will see other people as being thin. I'm different; I also view other people as being fat, even if they aren't. If someone says that so-and-so is thin, I will frequently think otherwise.

I say this is an interesting observation, because it suggests that somehow my feelings of being fat don't stem from some personal issue (if they did, then I'd think others were skinny), but from some kind of misconception as to what skinny or fat really is. I'm not saying that I never see a person who I think is skinny. I'm merely suggesting that I may have an overly strict definition of what it means to be thin.

In this chapter, I've told you about my early years. I felt fat, but that's it. I thought about dieting, but never actually went on one–at least not for more than a couple of days. I don't know if this was due to a lack of willpower or what. After the next chapter, I will tell you about how my problems really began.

Chapter 3

My Parents

Before I go any further, I would like to take a break from talking about myself, and tell you about two very special people, my parents, Jerry and Gail. Let's start with my dad.

To my father, who was a salesman, family was everything. I speak in the past tense, because my dad died in July 1988 after an eighteen-month battle with amyotrophic lateral sclerosis (ALS), also known as Lou Gehrig's disease.

Dad and I did all the usual father-and-son activities, but I'd be willing to bet that he spent more time and energy on these activities than other fathers did. Why did he do this? Because he'd have just as good a time as I would. Dad, however, derived more satisfaction from seeing me enjoy these activities than from participating in them himself. A perfect example is my old hobby, comic books. Up until 1984, when I quit collecting, I had accumulated about two or three thousand comic books. My favorite memories of my father are of the times we spent on my collection. He would drive me all over Massachusetts to different stores and conventions, not because he was fond of comic books, but because he knew how much I enjoyed them.

My mother and father shared similar values. Throughout this book, you will see just how much family means to her, especially as shown in how she has put up with me. Mom was the one who would do all the things for me that I did not see as important at the time, but looking back, now realize they were—getting me ready for school in the morning, helping me with my homework, driving me anywhere I needed or wanted to go, etc., etc. She was the one who kept the family in line.

It is impossible to tell you about everything my parents did. Among other things, they participated in the parents' groups of my public school and my temple. My mom was president of the PTA and volunteered in the school library. One year, my dad coached my Little League baseball team. I remember constantly teasing him about his great success as a coach. We had a perfect record—lost all eighteen games.

I think my parents' feelings about their children can best be summed up by saying that they never missed a single event, be it sporting, theatrical, intellectual, or otherwise—important or unimportant—in which Neil or I participated. They were always there, always supporting us.

Chapter 4

Troubles Begin

It was at the start of my first year in high school, September 1983, that my "fat feelings" gained strength, and my troubles started. Oddly, it was strange behavior of a different sort that preceded the anorexia. As a freshman, I became obsessed with studying. It did not really start out as an obsession; I just had a strong desire to do well. Sure, I studied more than the average student, but nothing too out of the ordinary. The praise I received from my parents and teachers gave me a great deal of pleasure and made me feel very good about myself.

On the very first day of school, I signed up to run on the cross-country track team. I was an okay runner. I improved a lot after that first day.

In the middle of October, my grandfather died after suffering from cancer for about two years. As a young child, I had been very close with my Zayde (Yiddish for grandfather), but as I got older, I believe we grew apart. Everyone—family and doctors—would later say that his death had a lot to do with my problems. I say otherwise, but what do I know? Everyone else knows what I think better than I do. Who am I to say how I feel? It's true that his death coincided with the time that my depression and obsessive studying began, but as far as I'm concerned, it was just coincidence.

When the depression began, I quit the cross-country track team. I simply did not have the motivation. A month later, I tried out for and made the freshman basketball team. I sat on the bench 99 percent of the time and after about one month, my depression increased and the studying began to get out of hand. I quit basketball (I had already given up my newspaper route) and began to devote all my time to my school work.

I got home from school about 2:30 in the afternoon and studied until midnight. Soon, I was studying until 1:00 in the morning—then 2:00. Eventually, I started going to bed at 2:00 a.m. and setting my alarm for 4:00 a.m., so that I could study some more before school. I even studied on the fifteen-minute bus ride to school.

I had friends, but my social life greatly decreased, and I allowed myself only an occasional break, usually on Friday nights. My parents and I would go out to dinner, and then spend the evening together. These evenings were really nice, even if all we did was watch television. The enjoyment came from just being together and relaxing. I had managed to continue my comic book collection. One Saturday each month, I would spend the day with my father at a comic book store or convention. However, the depression and studying soon started to interfere with the hobby I had loved so much. I lost interest, and eventually stopped collecting comic books.

The studying was probably part obsession, part perfection. Every piece of homework had to be immaculate. For instance, my math homework could not have one little erasure mark. This meant I might have to copy it over four, five, or six times. This perfection was very frustrating. To vent this frustration, I began banging my head against the wall.

I have been rambling on about my obsessiveness, but I really have not made it clear why I was studying so much. Most people would tell me, "Just put the books away and do something else." However, I wasn't able to. My parents pleaded with me to stop being so obsessed and to get some sleep, but I just couldn't. My mind was stuck on studying. I felt very guilty for not studying, as if it were wrong for me not to.

During these few months that my studying and depression worsened, I began to see a psychiatrist, Dr. C. A few years earlier, Dr. Alan Nauss, my pediatrician since I was about two years old, had recommended Dr. C to my parents when my father and brother were having difficulty getting along and were always arguing. After only two sessions, Dr. C suggested that these arguments were the result of mood swings Neil was having, which were caused by a medication he was taking for allergies. As soon as the medication was stopped, the fighting ended, and everything was fine. Because of what he had done for our family, my parents and I held Dr. C in very high esteem. To us, doctors were miracle workers. We had the incorrect belief that when you go to a doctor with your problem, he can solve it with a snap of his fingers.

When I first started seeing Dr. C–it was around December–I was extremely optimistic. I had no experience with mental illness. I figured that after a couple of meetings, Dr. C would say that such and such a thing was the matter, and then offer a solution. This didn't happen. Dr. C did not have any quick answers for my case.

Despite not having any success with Dr. C, I remained hopeful. I was full of questions and willing to do anything he suggested. I was seeing him once a week, on Saturdays, because I was too busy studying during the week. At each session I asked him, "What can I do to help myself? What do you suggest I do? How about if I try this or that?" At my request, my parents even took me to a hypnotist, Dr. Q.

I thought that if I were hypnotized, maybe I would be able to say why I felt the need to study so much, and why I felt guilty when I didn't study. I had only two meetings with Dr. Q. As it turned out, my lack of concentration, which increased with the depression, made me a noncandidate for hypnosis.

Dr. C prescribed antidepressant medication. From 1984 until 1990, I was on and off different antidepressants (nortriptyline, imipramine, desipramine, amoxapine, amitriptyline, and Prozac). Since none of these ever helped or made any difference, there is no point in discussing each time I began a new one. Some were stopped because of side effects, such as drowsiness, lightheadedness, fidgetiness (the most bothersome–like the jitters), and uncontrollable shaking. Others were stopped because they had no effect one way or the other.

In April 1984, I was getting a maximum of two hours sleep a

night. My parents and Dr. C decided to withdraw me from school. They made the right decision. Deep down, I think I wanted this to happen. By being out of school, I did not have the need to study. There was nothing I could do about it. Because I had no control over the matter, I would not feel guilty for not studying. Once I was out of school, it was out of my hands.

I was now seeing Dr. C three times a week, and I believe he made the right decision to remove me from school. As I look back, however, I think he may have been responsible for what happened next, but I'm not sure. Actually, no one is really to blame. Perhaps what happened next was inevitable. In any case, I should hold myself accountable for my own actions. It's just that I think Dr. C put the idea into my mind. Let me try to explain.

When he took me out of school, Dr. C said that he had one main concern. He was worried that I would replace my obsession with studying with a new obsession. This possibility had never occurred to me until he mentioned it. Dr. C put the idea of a new obsession into my mind. As a result, when I left school, I found myself thinking, "Okay, Dr. C said I might end up with a new obsession; now, what can I do to replace the studying?" In other words, I made a conscious effort to find a new obsession. To this day, although I could be wrong, I truly believe that this would not have happened if Dr. C had not said anything.

What was this new obsession? It was toothbrushing. At first, I was brushing about two hours per day. Very soon, it was twelve hours per day. While either sitting in front of the television or walking around the house, I would brush, brush, brush. This lasted for only a couple of weeks (I went through a lot of toothpaste and a lot of toothbrushes), before I made the decision that would lead to the anorexia.

I really hated the toothbrushing. Who wouldn't? One day, I woke up and said to myself, "Oh, gee, I don't want to brush my teeth all day. Well, hey, don't have anything to eat, your mouth won't get dirty, and you won't have to brush." With this in mind,

I didn't eat that day. I also did not eat (I did drink water) for the next three days.

Of course, Dr. C and my parents became extremely worried about my physical well-being. Finally, on June 16, I was admitted to Westwood Lodge, a psychiatric hospital in Westwood, Massachusetts. Westwood was almost like a vacation resort, complete with basketball court and swimming pool. It had a locked ward and an unlocked ward. Upon admittance, everyone was assigned to the locked unit for observation for a minimum of twenty-four hours. Depending upon one's condition, a patient may be transferred to the unlocked ward after this initial period, or remain on the locked ward for months.

Upon being admitted, I was assigned to Dr. B. He was now the boss. I was through with Dr. C. I still refused to have anything but water. My vital signs became very bad. My blood pressure was so low that the nurse had trouble taking it. My temperature was below 96 degrees. When reclining, my pulse would be 60, but would go up to 170 as soon as I stood. After four days (I had gone a total of eight days with nothing but water—the four days before the hospital and the four days in the hospital), I was given the following option: The next morning, June 21, I could have 500 calories, or I could be sent to a medical hospital to be force-fed. I ate that morning. I really tried. However, I had only about 400 calories, and I was discharged with instructions that I should be taken to a medical facility.

My parents decided to stop first and see Dr. Nauss. To this day, I don't know why Dr. B was not satisfied. Perhaps he wanted to immediately impress upon me that he was in control. ("I'm the boss. If I say 500 calories, then it will be 500 calories—not 400—period.") Maybe he had some other reason. I don't know, but I think he could have been a bit more flexible. Sure, I had not consumed the required amount, but I had tried. I mean, come on.

Subsequently, Dr. Nauss said that if I went home and ate, the force-feeding would not be necessary. I did what he said. During the five days I was home, Dr. Nauss kept in touch with me by phone and made sure I was eating. On June 25, I returned to Westwood Lodge.

My program at Westwood was simple. I had three meals per day. After each meal, I was given my toothbrush for fifteen minutes. At all other times, my toothbrush was kept by the staff. I met with Dr. B daily and attended group, adolescent, music, and occupational therapy. My parents and I were assigned to a social worker, Ms. T, with whom we met on a weekly basis. I spent most of my free time at occupational therapy, where I made paper-towel holders, napkin holders, hot-plate holders, and other novelties. I even had a small crush on one of the aides working there. In the evenings, patients and staff would play different board games, the most popular being Trivial Pursuit.

Based on their progress, patients were given privileges–for example, being allowed to walk unaccompanied on hospital grounds. The highest level of privileges, which I had after about one month, was permission to leave the hospital with the staff to go bowling or to the movies. Before being discharged from the hospital, a patient might be granted "passes" to leave the hospital for a couple of hours–sometimes overnight–with family or friends.

My feelings about the hospital were similar to those I had when I was taken out of school. Deep down, I think that I wanted to be hospitalized. It was a relief. Again, it was a control issue. I had to eat–I thought I had no choice (in later years, I would realize that I had more control than I thought), but I couldn't brush my teeth more than the allotted fifteen minutes. I would not feel guilty for not brushing because I had no control over it.

After a few weeks, the toothbrushing was no longer a problem. There was really no explanation for this. I think it was simply a matter of "out of sight, out of mind." Fifteen minutes after each meal just became a way of life. I was soon allowed to keep my own toothbrush and transferred to the unlocked ward.

Westwood was the only hospital at which I made friends–or even talked–with the staff or other patients. At any given time, there would be between five and ten adolescents. However, even though I was only fifteen years old, I was always more comfortable around the adults.

This was my first time around "sick" or "crazy" or "weird" people. However, contrary to popular belief, these people were not out of their minds. They were your average, everyday people, who were merely having some personal trouble. Other adolescents were there because they did not get along with their parents, had developed a smoking or alcohol problem, or were depressed. The adults were there for many different reasons. Depression, smoking or alcohol addiction, marital difficulties, and other family problems were the most common reasons. As I said, there was nothing "wrong" with these people. A lot of people have similar problems. These individuals just had them to a greater degree and were looking for some help.

How does everything I've been telling you about Westwood and the toothbrushing relate to the anorexia? Well, as you know, I'd been feeling fat for years, but never believed that I had the willpower to diet. Now, I saw that I did. The anorexia became the focus of my life.

I always believed that feeling fat was something I couldn't help. This was no longer the case. There was something I could do about it. I had the willpower to diet. I was all-powerful Michael. No longer would I feel fat and put up with it. Instead, I would do something or hate myself. Except for my family, Dr. B was the first person to whom I ever mentioned feeling fat. When I did this, he told me it was a characteristic of anorexia nervosa. "What's that?" I asked. When he explained the condition, I automatically labeled myself an anorexic. It's hard to explain, but it almost seemed "glamorous" to me (I don't know if that's the right word), something I wanted. I had an illness; I had something few others had; I was special. The anorexia gave me an identity and made me an individual.

It was at Westwood that I first became focused on the weight (number of pounds) itself. At one point, I was weighing myself hourly or every other hour. This did not last long. There was no point in constant weight checking. There would be basically no change.

The first way I noticed a difference in my weight was that my clothes felt loose. This made me feel *so* good. For the next five or six years, whenever I would be losing weight, I would get a "high" by getting dressed in the morning, and feeling that my pants had become that much bigger on me.

After being at Westwood for two months, my insurance ran out. There was really no reason for me not to go home. The toothbrushing wasn't a problem, and although I thought of losing weight, this had not yet become a serious issue. However, Dr. B and I did have one concern about my going home. It was mid-August, about three weeks before the start of school. We feared that in an unstructured environment, with a lot of free time on my hands, I would fall back into the habit of brushing my teeth. Because of this, it was decided that I would be transferred to the psychiatric ward of Norwood Hospital, a medical facility in Norwood, Massachusetts. (Insurance would not cover my stay at a private psychiatric hospital, but it would cover my stay on a psychiatric ward of a medical hospital.) I would stay there for about two weeks and go home one week before school started. This week would give me time to get back into the flow of everyday life outside the hospital.

In essence, Norwood was just "temporary housing" for me, noteworthy for only one reason. It was here that I had my first feelings of competition. There were one or two other anorexics (there had been none at Westwood). I felt that I had to be the skinniest, lose more weight than anyone else, and have the strictest guidelines around what I did or did not eat. These feelings were not strong, nor did I act on them. However, they were there.

Chapter 5

Back to School

When I returned home from the hospital the last week in August, I did not keep the anorexia a secret. When I had left school in April, I had said that it was because of mononucleosis. At the time, the other students knew that I studied a lot, but they did not know to what degree. The idea of seeing a psychiatrist, and later of being in a psychiatric hospital, had embarrassed me. I now knew that there was no reason for this embarrassment. Others could accept me as I was or shun me. It was their choice.

Some of the students were understanding. Some thought I was joking. Some didn't care one way or the other. Some shied away because they were uneasy and not sure of what to say or do or think. This was understandable; it wasn't as though they had a lot of experience in the matter. Actually, there was no reason to treat me any differently. I wasn't abnormal; I merely had a few problems. Still others openly ignored and stayed away from me because I was "weird." After all, I was seeing a shrink and had spent two months in a "sicko" hospital.

Before my discharge from Westwood, Dr. B, my parents, and I had set a program I was to follow outside of the hospital. I needed to maintain my weight at 120 pounds, which was what it had been during my hospitalization. (I don't remember how much I had weighed before the hospital–maybe around 135.) Anything less would put me in serious medical danger and require rehospitalization, perhaps even tube feeding. This is a perfect example of why I now ignore doctors and believe that half the time, they don't know what they're talking about. Anything less than 120 pounds would be medically dangerous, and yet here I am today, not in great shape but functioning okay, at 75 pounds.

In addition to the weight maintenance, I would continue to brush my teeth three times a day for fifteen minutes each time, go to bed by midnight, and participate in an extracurricular activity. Dr. B also recommended, and arranged for me to see, Dr. J, another psychiatrist. My parents and I had wanted me to continue with Dr. B, but he already had a full schedule.

On my first day back at school, I once again signed up for the cross-country track team. This would be my extracurricular activity. However, two days later, I quit. I was still depressed and just didn't have the motivation. Instead of a school-related activity, I got a part-time job. I worked approximately ten hours a week in the public library as a library page.

For the first few months of school, which were from September 1984 until the beginning of 1985, things remained basically the same. I was seeing Dr. P two times a week and sticking to the agreement I had made upon leaving Westwood. Around the beginning of 1985, things began to go downhill.

Chapter 6

Five Unusual Habits

My depression led to a lack of interest in socializing and other people. Soon, I had no friends and no social life. Some of my old friends remained faithful and let it be known that they would always be there for me, but I didn't really care.

I lost five pounds, going down to 115. I take complete responsibility for my actions, the weight loss was my own doing. However, perhaps by not taking any action, Dr. P allowed me to think that I could get away with losing weight whenever I felt like it. I am not saying this is the case. Maybe it wasn't, since I did maintain the 115 for a year or so, but. . .

In addition to the continuous depression, which had increased since my return to school, and the weight loss, I developed some unusual habits, which I still follow. The five most prevalent were (1) refusal to eat any low-calorie or diet foods, (2) refusal to let anyone see me eat, (3) constant wearing of jacket or bathrobes, (4) refusal to drink water, and (5) refusal to swallow my saliva.

(1) *Refusal to eat any low-calorie or diet foods.* I don't know if they are right, but this, along with the refusal to drink water, is a characteristic of mine that has led various therapists to label me as one of the most severe anorexics they have ever encountered. Many anorexics will allow themselves to fill up on low-calorie foods (diet sodas, salads, etc.), so that they will not be hungry. To me, this demonstrates a lack of willpower. I will not let myself fill up on these foods. Abstinence is the key to my feelings of self-control and being all-powerful–almost as though restricting my intake is a challenge.

(2) *Refusal to let anyone see me eat.* Aside from my mother

and brother, I will not eat in front of anyone. I first became uneasy in the school cafeteria. I felt that the other students were watching me, as if I were a pig. I started thinking, "Gee, they're probably wondering what I'm doing with food. After all, I have anorexia–I'm not supposed to eat." It was probably my imagination; they most likely never even noticed me. Odds are, none of them could have cared less. Still, I was uncomfortable and decided from then on to have my lunch in the bathroom, a private cubicle in the library, or anywhere else I wouldn't be seen. This carried over into my house. If we had guests, they did not see me eat.

(3) *Constant wearing of jacket or bathrobes.* Because I feel fat whenever I look at myself, I always wear a jacket in public to cover up my stomach. I don't mean occasionally, but almost all the time. When I am home, I will wear two bathrobes instead of the jacket, taking them off only when I go to bed or shower. I know that when I was in school, some of the students considered me strange because of my depression and unsociability. I don't know what they thought of my constant need to wear a jacket, but it probably added to my "weird" image. With one or two exceptions, since graduation, I haven't seen any of the kids from school. Maybe some of them are reading this book right now, thinking, "I remember that loser. So that's why he never took off his coat."

(4) *Refusal to drink water.* I do not drink water–I mean never. I have not had any water since February 1985. Now, I know there is water in everything. What I mean by no water is that I will not drink plain water; I will not go to a sink, pour myself some water, and drink it. This coincides with what I said earlier about my refusal to have any low-calorie or diet foods. The abstinence from water is almost like a challenge. I know water has no calories, but I would still feel fat if I drank it.

I remember the day I decided to stop drinking water. I had worked at the library from six in the evening until nine. I got home about fifteen minutes later, and ran to the sink to gulp down a few glasses of water. This was something I frequently did. With my dry mouth, a side effect of antidepressant medication and a result of limited intake, I was usually thirsty. After I had the water, I lifted my shirt, looked at my stomach, and felt so fat. I saw my stomach as sticking out, immensely bloated. I decided right then and there that I would never again drink water. If I was thirsty, that would be my tough luck. Talk about will-power. I have not had a drink of water since.

(5) *Refusal to swallow my saliva.* In March, a month after I stopped having water, I decided not to swallow my saliva. This is stupid, you say? I know. I agree. But, it's the way I am. I constantly spit out my saliva. To do this, I always have a paper cup or a paper towel in my jacket pocket. I spit into these twenty-four hours per day. Even when I go to sleep in the evening, I keep one or the other by my side.

Chapter 7

The Silent Psychiatrist

Let me tell you a bit about Dr. P. As I said, Dr. B recommended him at the time of my discharge from Westwood Lodge. I saw Dr. P two times a week; each session lasted fifty minutes. For the first few months, I looked forward to our meetings. I wanted to get better and was willing to do anything. I guess I still thought of doctors as being miracle workers. This soon changed with Dr. P.

I began to see our meetings as a waste of my time and my parents' money. The depression continued to grow. I lost my desire to get better and was soon wishing that I were dead. Dr. P was almost always late, usually by thirty to forty-five minutes. One time, he was almost one and a half hours late. "My time's as important as yours," I told him. "When you're late, I have to wait in the reception area by myself. There's no receptionist or anything. For all I know, you've forgotten about the appointment and aren't even going to show up. Occasionally being a little late is one thing, but. . . Next time you're late, I'm leaving. And we won't pay for that appointment." A week or so later, he was late, and I left. At our next meeting, I told him not to bother sending a bill for that missed session. Sure enough, he was never again late.

What were our sessions like? Well, a typical session would start with each of us saying hello. Then we would sit down and look at each other. After doing this for fifty minutes, he would tell me that my time was up, and I would leave. This is the truth. I'm serious. He was getting paid around sixty dollars per hour, and we were staring at each other. That's all. No talking. I think I even occasionally dozed off (sixty dollars is an expensive nap).

In all, I saw Dr. P for almost two and a half years; our sessions came to an end when he moved to another state. During this time, my depression increased to the point where it could not get any worse. It never let up. I just wanted to die.

I frequently told my parents that I wanted to stop seeing Dr. P. He did not help and was a complete waste of time. I could be wrong, but I believe he was more interested in money than anything else (either that, or he was totally incompetent).

Because I felt that Dr. P was not helping, my parents sought the advice of Dr. B and other doctors whom they knew. However, all these doctors recommended that I continue to see Dr. P, and therefore, I did. Although I had become more depressed and lost a little weight, my parents did not know what else to do. Perhaps they feared that if I stopped seeing Dr. P, I would "fall apart." My parents were doing what they thought was best, maybe entertaining some false hope about what I could get out of these doctor appointments.

Although concern about anorexia is growing, there is still a large unawareness, especially about male anorexia, and this is the major purpose of my story—so that other men with this problem will realize that they are not alone. My parents and I could not pick up a book and read about male anorexics. For all we knew, I was the only man in the world with anorexia. My parents did not know how to deal with me or even what to think. We had no one to whom we could turn. Perhaps if a book like this one had been around at the time, things would have been different.

Chapter 8

A Well-Kept Secret

During the summer of 1985, between my sophomore and junior years of high school, I had two part-time jobs. I continued working at the library, and also worked as a teacher's aide at a camp in my temple's nursery school.

My junior year started in September 1985. At the beginning of 1986, I stopped having lunch (this had been nothing more than a dry bologna-and-cheese sandwich; I didn't even have anything to drink with it). I had been eating three times a day, but now I would eat only twice, once in the morning and once in the evening. I can't say for sure exactly what led to this decision. It probably had to do with my need to feel in control. By not having lunch, I was practicing even more abstinence.

This was also the time I did something that I have never told anyone about until now. I was well aware of how bad my parents felt about the anorexia. So often, I felt guilty about what I put them through. If anyone deserved to be happy, they did. I wanted to do something–anything–for them. I don't mean simply buying a gift and giving it to them. I wanted to do something that had meaning to it.

One Sunday, they planned to drive to Cape Cod for the day. Before they left, I went into my mother's purse and took the key to our family's other car off her key ring. Keep in mind, I was a couple of months short of my seventeenth birthday and did not yet have my driver's license.

After they left, I took the car and drove to four different bakeries. My intention was to get some cupcakes and juice, and to sit down and eat my dinner with my parents. It had been a while since we had sat down together at the table (I ate standing over the kitchen counter). I was sure that dinner together would be special. Although the cupcakes and juice would cost only a couple of dollars, this was a perfect example of the saying, "When giving a gift, it's the thought that counts." This would have more meaning than an expensive gift—it really came from the heart.

Why so many bakeries? Well, each time I was about to buy something, I would start feeling fat, become aggravated and full of self-doubt, and would leave without the cupcakes. At the fourth bakery, I finally bought the cupcakes, then went to the market and purchased some juice.

Because I went to so many bakeries, this little errand took me almost the entire day. By the time I got home, I was tired and frustrated. I hated myself for making such an issue of the whole thing and not simply buying something at the first bakery. When I thought of actually eating the cupcakes, I felt fat. The result? After all this, I just threw everything away, went upstairs to my room, yelled at myself for being such a jerk and a lousy son, and banged my head against the wall to vent my frustration.

As I said, this is the one episode I've always kept secret. I never even told my parents. Maybe they had some way of finding out and knew what I had done. It's possible, but I don't think so. When my mother reads this, I don't know what her reaction will be. It happened such a long time ago, she probably won't have any feelings one way or the other.

Well, Mom, what do you think?

Chapter 9

The Refrigerator Experiment

The routine of my life remained the same throughout my junior year. I went to school, worked at the library, studied (I still studied a lot, but it was not an obsession), and went to bed. I had no interests whatsoever, no social life, and not even one friend.

I don't know what my teachers thought of me. Scholastically speaking, I know they believed I was a very good student and a hard worker. I don't know what their opinions of me as a person were. They may have thought I was unusual or strange or different. They may not have thought anything at all.

In gym class, the teachers were extremely lenient. Students did not receive a letter grade, just a pass or fail mark. In order to pass, all that was necessary was to show up with shorts and a T-shirt, ready to participate. However, you did not actually have to participate. At least, I didn't. I would be in my shorts and T-shirt (and jacket to cover myself), but would just sit and watch the others. This was fine with me. I was not overly strong. Along with the depression and lack of motivation, I probably would not have been able to participate anyway.

For all I know, I may have been permitted not to do anything because my parents or doctor had intervened and made some arrangement with the school—it's possible, but I doubt it. I don't think Dr. P would have had the initiative, but I don't know everything. I'm the first to say that I could be wrong. Maybe the instructors felt sorry for me. Perhaps they were afraid that if I participated, I would collapse, and they decided it was best not to take this chance. Again, these are possibilities, but I don't think so. At this time, although I was skinny, I don't believe that I looked emaciated. I'm probably reading too much into my teachers' leniency. It's completely possible that they were just easygoing or simply did not care.

About the middle of 1986, at my suggestion, I got my own refrigerator. Here's the story.

Every so often, perhaps once a month or every couple of months, Dr. P, my parents, and I would have a family meeting. There was conversation at these meetings—no silent-psychiatrist routine. My parents' hopes never ended. They were full of questions and ideas. Dr. P probably decided he had to appear both interested and competent, because my parents paid his bills.

At one of these meetings, my parents mentioned that they were worried about what would happen after I graduated from high school. If I went away to college or just out on my own, what would my life be like? What would happen in terms of the depression? How would the food issue be handled?

Well, we agreed that with my grades, I would most likely go on to college. "If I live in a college dorm, I'll just fend for myself," I said. "Of course, a meal plan would be a waste of money. I eat so little, it would be cheaper for me to get by on my own, instead of with college food. Since I won't eat in front of anyone, a dorm would have to be a single. Most colleges don't allot these to freshmen, so I'll most likely end up in an off-campus efficiency."

Whether an efficiency or a private room in a dorm, I would end up being responsible for my own food. A strong possibility was that I'd have my own refrigerator—a small one, similar to what many college students have in their dorms. "Why not have a test run, now? We could get the refrigerator, keep it in the basement, and I'll act as though I'm in college," I suggested.

Although I added that I could manage fine without a refrigerator, my parents said they'd feel better if I had one, and we ended up getting it. I had received my driver's license and was now responsible for my own food affairs. Once a week, I would drive to the market and get my own food.

At first, I felt I had to prove to myself that I could get by on only a few dollars, as well as without any refrigerator at all. I refused to spend more than $3.00 per week and ended up having a lot of stale bread and warm soda. After this initial self-test period of about a month, I was willing to use the refrigerator and stopped paying attention to prices.

Looking back, I think I suggested the refrigerator for myself, as well as to show my parents that I could manage. The depression, of course, was always present. I still had no interests and pretty much no life, aside from school and work. The market gave me something to do, something "to look forward to." It also gave me a sense of freedom and independence.

Chapter 10

My Odyssey

My junior year ended, and that summer I had two jobs. I was still at the library for ten or fifteen hours a week. I also started working forty hours a week as a cashier in a supermarket. Not bad for someone supposedly in such poor physical health.

At the beginning of my senior year, September 1986, I left my job at the library and continued working part-time at the supermarket.

At the beginning of 1987, my family was struck with horrible news. Lately, my father had not been feeling well. There was nothing specifically wrong; he was just unhealthy in general. He had fallen once, but we thought he had just slipped on the ice. We were wrong. He fell again, and this time, he broke his ankle. This led to some tests. On January 15, my father was diagnosed with amyotrophic lateral sclerosis (ALS), a form of muscular dystrophy. My father was dying. There was no cure, nothing that could be done. He might live for twenty years, or only one year; in any event, he would not get better.

My father dealt with this news, at least in terms of his outward demeanor, better than most people would have. His way of coping was to joke. "Maybe I can be a poster boy for the Jerry Lewis Telethon" was his favorite quip. He was determined to live his life to the fullest and to enjoy the time he had left, not lament or feel sorry for himself.

I swear to you, he was one of the greatest.

The rest of my senior year was uneventful. I applied to only one college, Babson College in Wellesley, Massachusetts, and was accepted under the early admissions program. Since this was only about a thirty-minute drive from Framingham, my parents and I decided that I would live at home and commute. I applied to only one school, because I did not care whether or not I attended college at all. I went only because my parents wanted me to–I was trying to please them.

Midway through my senior year, around February 1987, Dr. P moved to Vermont or Virginia–I'm not sure which. Of course, I was very disappointed to see him leave, since he meant so much to me. Seriously speaking, good riddance. I temporarily was not seeing anyone, which was fine with me, when another psychiatrist, Dr. D, was recommended to us. At my parents' request, I began seeing him on a regular basis.

Remember my escapade at the bakeries? Well, I tried it again at the beginning of June, and was successful. I did not make a big deal about it; I simply went to one place and bought the food. That evening, my parents and I sat down and ate our dinners together for the first time since late 1984. It was even more special because it came around the time of their anniversary, which was June 7.

Upon graduating high school in June, I returned to the library. Now that I had my diploma, I was able to work as a library assistant. I spent the summer working there part-time and also part-time at the supermarket. When college began, I left my job as a supermarket cashier and continued working part-time at the library.

I started college in September 1987. This was my "excuse" for losing weight. I had already started to lose weight sometime during my junior and senior years in high school (not much–just a few pounds). I don't recall exactly when. Now that I was commuting to college, I stayed in bed late, and when I got up, I skipped breakfast, claiming that I did not have the time. Of course, this was just a cop-out. I intentionally stayed in bed, awake, for two or three hours, so that when I did get up, I really didn't have the time to eat.

Soon, I was skipping breakfast more often than I was having it, and my weight really began to drop. I didn't even bother to create an excuse by staying in bed late. I would get up early and just decide not to eat. Skipping breakfast meant that I would be eating only one meal a day–dinner. My parents were extremely worried. This was the first time that they actually yelled at me over the food issue.

The weight loss got out of control. I had lost about 15 or 20 pounds and was down to around 96. On October 29, Dr. D had me admitted to the psychiatric unit of Emerson Hospital in Concord, Massachusetts.

While I was at Emerson, my parents visited me every day, even though this was difficult for my dad, who by this time was in a wheelchair. There is nothing else I can tell you about my stay at Emerson. I just don't remember anything. However, I do remember what happened the day I left the hospital.

Dr. D, the staff, and I made an agreement that when I went above 100 pounds, I could leave the hospital during the day to attend classes at Babson. This meant approximately a 5-pound weight gain. Permission to leave the hospital would be my reward for gaining weight. It was supposed to supply me with an incentive. Instead, the exact opposite happened. At this time, I decided to kill myself. I had thought about it in the past, and the time had come.

Now, I was (and still am) too much of a coward to shoot or stab myself or anything like that. The only way I would commit suicide is to fast and starve myself to death.

I pretended to be very enthusiastic about our agreement. However, in the back of my mind, I was thinking, "Let them believe you're willingly increasing your weight. Just gain the 4 or 5 pounds so you can have a chance to get out of here." My plan was to leave the hospital, take off somewhere–anywhere–and starve myself to death.

I gained the 5 pounds. The established protocol was weight gain of 1/2 pound per day. I accomplished this only by constantly reminding myself, "It's only for a week or so. Gain the weight–it's only 4 or 5 pounds–and then you can take off."

On November 9, about one and a half weeks after my admission to Emerson, I reached the 100-pound "goal." That morning, my mother picked me up at the hospital and dropped me off at Babson College. However, I did not go to my classes. I had never intended to. Instead, I took the bus from the college to my bank in Framingham. I withdrew some money, went to the Greyhound bus station in Boston, and bought a one-way ticket to Orlando, Florida.

My mother was supposed to pick me up at Babson around noon. I called home and lied. "I have to stay later than I thought," I said. "I called the hospital, and they said it would be okay. I'm not sure how long I'll be, so I'll call you later."

I had decided to starve myself to death. I was not going to put a single thing in my mouth. I mean absolutely nothing.

While I was away that week, my parents did all they could to find me. They had the police looking for me and even hired a private detective. There were also articles in the newspaper, and a $1,000 cash reward. (See Figure 10.1.) I kept a small diary during this trip. Instead of trying to jog my memory as to what happened during this time, I think it would be better if I just reproduced the diary.

*   *   *

Monday, November 9. At 8:30 a.m., I take the bus from Babson to the bank. After taking out some money, I go to the Greyhound bus station. About 12:30 p.m., I call home. My mom was going to pick me up in the early afternoon to take me back to the hospital. I tell her that I need to stay later than I expected, that I had called the hospital and been given permission, and that I would call later when I was done. At 2:45 p.m., I buy a ticket to Orlando, Florida. The bus doesn't leave until 4:00 p.m. I spend half an hour walking around downtown Boston. Then, I call my parents to let them know that I'm leaving. I'm going to starve myself to death (this diary is being written for them; I know they'll have some interest in knowing what I've done; furthermore, many doctors may find my story interesting). The bus arrives in New York City at 9:20 p.m. Bus doesn't leave until 10:00 p.m. I call my parents (they tell me the police are looking for me, and that they've hired a private detective) and miss my bus. Next bus isn't until 11:15 p.m. If I sit down, I might get mugged; I pass the time by walking around outside.

FIGURE 10.1

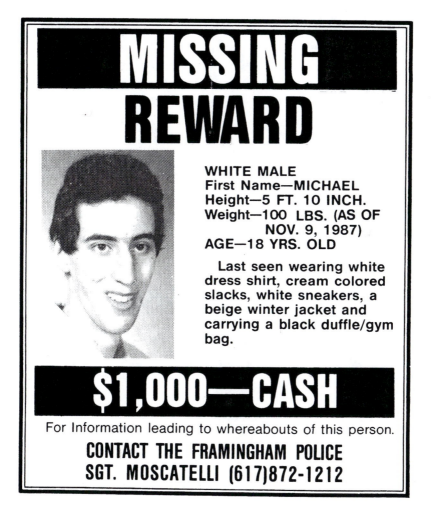

From the *Middlesex News*, November 11, 1987. (Reprinted by permission of *Middlesex News*, Framingham, Massachusetts.)

Tuesday, November 10. From 11:15 p.m., Monday, to 10:15 p.m., Tuesday, I'm on the bus. We make thirty-minute stops in Virginia, North Carolina, South Carolina, and a few other places. I either remain on the bus, call my parents, or browse through the gift shop. By the way, my handwriting is not messy because I'm "so weak and unhealthy." I am doing all this writing on the bus, which makes it difficult to be neat.

While in South Carolina, the police come on the bus—it's not for me. Instead, it is to remove some disorderly passengers.

I arrive in Jacksonville at 10:15 p.m. on Tuesday. The last time I ate was Sunday night at 5:00 (over fifty hours ago). I could continue to Orlando but would arrive at 2:10 a.m. I decide to spend the night in Jacksonville at the Econo Lodge. I arrive at the hotel around midnight and go right to bed.

Wednesday, November 11. I wake up around 7:00 a.m., check out of the hotel at 10:30, and arrive at the bus station at 11:15. The bus doesn't leave until 2:45, so I pass the time walking around downtown Jacksonville. I walk for two and half hours, nonstop. If I'm so weak, then I don't know how I'm able to do so much walking. I have done more walking since Monday morning than I can remember having done at all over the past few years.

During my two and a half hours of walking, I stop in Woolworth's. They have a coin-operated, digital scale. I have never trusted digital scales, especially ones that cost money, but I figure I'll weigh myself. I take off my jacket and sneakers. I'm in the same clothes that I always wear to weigh myself. At 1:00 p.m., I weigh 96.0 pounds. I leave Jacksonville at 2:45 and arrive in Orlando at 6:20 p.m. I still have not had anything since Sunday night (72 hours). According to what doctors have told me in the past, a person can go without food or water for five to ten days. I must be about halfway there. (NOTE: When I say that I have not had anything, this includes water; the last time I had a drink of water was February 1985.)

I feel the same now as I always have.

After arriving in Orlando, I walk to the Travelodge. I get there at 9:20 p.m. I don't know what I'm going to do tomorrow.

Thursday, November 12. I wake up a little before 8:00 a.m. and check out of the hotel at about 9:00. I take the shuttle to a mall and walk around for a couple of hours. My entire body is fine, except my legs feel very heavy (actually, it's my calves). Walking seems to be easier than standing. I could check into a hotel and just stay in Orlando for the next week, but I don't know how hard the police are looking for me. I have no idea if they've been able to trace me or if they have no clue whatsoever as to where I am. I guess I'll just keep on moving. I consider many options. I decide to take the Amtrak train back to Boston and take my chances with dying on the train. If I'm not dead when I get to Boston, I don't know what I'll do. I call my parents as usual. This time my mother asks the operator for time and charges.

When I hang up, I know the police are coming for me and that I should leave, but I don't. I don't know why, but I decide to play a waiting game and see if my train will leave before the police arrive. I was wrong. The police arrive. I've failed. My one mistake was letting my guilt about my parents overcome my better judgment.

Friday, November 13. I eat for the first time at 1:30 p.m. (about 116 hours without eating). Now, I know that I've really lost.

* * *

When I think about this trip, I don't know what my thoughts really are. Did I really want to die? Did I want to be found? Is this why I called my parents? Is this why I waited in the train station, even though I knew the police were on their way? I don't know. What I will say about those five days "on the run" is that I had peace of mind. I felt better about myself than I had for years. Yes, I felt guilty about what I was doing to my parents, but that's it. I didn't hate myself and just flat out felt at peace.

Chapter 11

More Hospitals

After the police picked me up at the train station, I was taken to Florida State Hospital. I do not remember anyone or anything from that hospital. All I know is that it was typical of everything you read and hear about state institutions—the bad conditions, poor treatment of patients, apathy on the part of the staff, etc., etc.

I was at Florida State for only two nights. The first night, I received intravenous (IV) fluids. An IV is used to feed a patient fluids through a needle in the arm.

After being contacted by the police and informed of my hospitalization, my mother and uncle (I have only one uncle, my mother's brother) flew down to get me. As it turned out, they had to go through a lot of red tape. For unknown reasons, the doctor assigned to me was hesitant to grant my release, and my mother had to contact the head of the hospital. Even then, the hospital would allow me to return to Massachusetts only if I went by air ambulance, which would cost about $8,000 ($8,000—can you believe it?). After what I had put everyone through, I should have been left at Florida State. I deserved it. However, my parents paid for the ambulance.

I have no idea what the purpose of the air ambulance was. What did we get for the money? Can you believe that they actually offered a small buffet dinner? A lot of good that was going to do me. A nurse took my vital signs, and that was it. Nothing else. Why couldn't we simply have bought three airline tickets?

On November 14, I returned to Massachusetts. Emerson Hospital did not want me back. The staff felt that they could not trust me. Therefore, I was taken to St. Elizabeth's Hospital in Brighton.

At St. Elizabeth's, I was on the locked unit of the psychiatric ward. I was admitted on a Section 12. This is the temporary commitment to a hospital (up to ten days) of a person who is considered to be a danger to himself or others. I soon signed a voluntary admission. My doctor during this three-week stay was a psychiatric resident, Dr. E. Upon admission, my pulse and blood pressure were average. However, my temperature was only 95 degrees. My weight was around 96 pounds.

I did not accomplish anything at St. Elizabeth's. I was weighed each day and maintained my weight, but that was it. I saw Dr. E daily. Otherwise, most of the time was spent just sitting around, maybe doing an occasional jigsaw puzzle. As always, my parents visited me every day.

Seeing my hospitalization as pointless, I submitted a three-day notice. The purpose of this notice is to give the doctor three days to go to court–if he chooses to–and show that I need to be committed because I am a danger to myself or others. Dr. E objected to my leaving the hospital, but did not fight it. I left St. Elizabeth's on December 4, AMA (Against Medical Advice). My weight was still 96 pounds.

Dr. E and I had gotten along well. I would have been willing to continue seeing her as an outpatient, but there was one hitch. My vital signs, especially my temperature, had been very low. Dr. E, who would be checking these vital signs each time I visited, said that if my temperature dropped below 96 degrees, I would need to return to the hospital. I was unwilling to see her as long as there was the possibility of rehospitalization. That was that, and I never again saw Dr. E.

Chapter 12

Back Home–Temporarily

During my stay at St. Elizabeth's, I had tried to keep the thought of starving myself to death out of my mind. Sometimes I was successful, sometimes not. Regardless, I knew, deep down, that it was only a matter of time.

Upon returning home, I went back to work. Because of my excellent grades, Babson had offered to put me on medical leave. However, I just didn't feel like going back to school. Instead, I returned to the library. Everyone there knew about me and what had happened, but if it bothered them, they did not let it show. They had always been kind to me, and I was welcomed back. Because the library was able to offer me only ten to twenty-five hours a week, I looked for a second part-time job. Through a friend of my mother's, I got one doing basic clerical work at a finance corporation.

For the next few months, my life was pretty routine. I woke up in the morning, showered, had breakfast, went to work or sat around the house, had dinner, watched TV or vegetated, and went to bed. As had been the case since high school, I did not have any social life or any kind of amusement. The depression was always there, and I simply had no interests.

As I said a couple of paragraphs back, I knew it was only a matter of time before something happened regarding my weight, and during these few months, while I was working, I was slowly losing weight–skipping or cutting back my breakfast or dinner (or both). Whether or not anyone knew or suspected what I was doing, I cannot say.

Upon leaving St. Elizabeth's the first week in December, I had weighed 96 pounds. On March 15, 1988, my weight was 81 pounds. I knew it could not go on much longer before someone did something, and on that day, I once again decided to run. That morning, my mother left to go to her uncle's funeral. I had written a couple of farewell notes (to my parents and Neil) and left them on my bed. I then walked across the street to the bank to get money for a bus ticket. I had not given much thought to leaving the notes out in the open. My father was home, but he was sleeping. Even if he had been awake, I don't think I would have thought twice about it, since I'd be gone for only thirty minutes.

Because of what had happened at Emerson, when I had taken money out in order to run, there was a restriction on my account. I was not supposed to be able to withdraw money from the bank. I knew that I would need a believable story to give the bank teller.

First, I reported that I had lost my bankbook and needed a new one. I left my old book in its usual location, my dresser drawer. Anyone checking my old book would not suspect that I had withdrawn any money.

After receiving a new bankbook, I asked to withdraw money. When the teller challenged this, I asked to see the manager. "The restriction was removed a while ago, and you should have a letter in your files authorizing this removal," I told the manager. "This is the third time I've had this trouble. I'm in a real rush and cannot wait. Maybe I'd be better off switching to another bank."

Probably because he was anxious to avoid any trouble, as well as eager to please a long-time customer (or because he simply did not care, and figured it wouldn't matter), the manager did not hesitate to give me my money.

Upon returning home from the bank, I found my father in hysterics. He had gone into my bedroom and found the notes. I have two opinions about this. One is that I just didn't think about leaving the notes on my bed or about the possibility my dad would find them. On the other hand, I can't help wondering if I left them there, hoping they would be found. This would coincide with my uncertainty about why I called home so often when

I ran to Orlando. Remember, I said that maybe I had called because I subconsciously hoped to be found—had remained in the train station, knowing that the police were coming, because I actually wanted to be caught. Well, perhaps leaving the notes where my dad could find them was my cry for help. I don't know.

Anyway, being helpless himself and not knowing what else to do, my dad called the funeral home, and my mother was paged in the middle of the ceremony. She returned shortly after I did. When my parents confronted me, I told them that I was not going to the hospital. I went so far as to take a knife and hold it to my chest. This was just a bluff. I've said that I would not have the courage to shoot or stab myself, or commit suicide by any means other than starvation.

My parents pleaded with me, and I gave them the knife. However, I still refused to go to the hospital. My mother immediately left, went to a friend of hers who worked in a psychiatrist's office, and got papers to have me committed.

Meanwhile, I began to suspect what she was doing and decided to take off. A little later, my mother returned with the commitment papers and an ambulance. However, I was not there, and the ambulance personnel would not do anything without the police. My brother, who had followed me to an apartment building, called to let everyone know where I was. The police came a bit later, and I "voluntarily" conceded. I was then taken to Bournewood Hospital in Brookline.

Chapter 13

Bournewood

It was at Bournewood Hospital that I met Dr. Stephen Wiener. Although I don't believe he could have helped me, this is my preconceived notion of all therapists. Because of my experiences with uncaring, incompetent doctors, I have a very low opinion of most of them. For a while now, I've said that no doctor is going to help make me better. Getting better is up to me–period. Perhaps if I had met Dr. Wiener three or four years earlier, when I wanted to get better and was willing, even anxious, to try anything, everything would have turned out differently. Maybe, maybe not. That's a question no one can answer.

Of all the doctors I have seen in my life, I think kindly about three of them: Dr. Nauss, Dr. Wiener, and Dr. Spielberg, whom you'll meet later. I believe they cared about me. I'm sure they cared about the money also–they had every right to. However, I feel that other doctors cared more about the money than me. I could be wrong, but I believe Drs. Nauss, Wiener, and Spielberg cared about me first. I'd go so far as to bet that if my family had been poor and unable to pay them, they still would have seen me. As I said, they cared about Michael Krasnow.

Although I had "voluntarily" gone to Bournewood with the police (I really had not been in any position to argue with them), I soon decided not to stay. On March 17, two days after my admission to Bournewood, I said I was leaving AMA and signed a three-day notice.

Dr. Wiener decided to take me to court to have me committed. I stated my case to the judge, who said I spoke very well, but that because of my appearance, he could not let me go and still live with himself. Therefore, on March 21, I was committed to Bournewood.

Bournewood was a psychiatric hospital, similar in some ways to Westwood Lodge, but not as luxurious. There were no swimming pools, basketball courts, or "field trips" to the movies. I remained there for about one month, the entire time spent on the locked ward. This ward consisted of two units, one male and one female. The male unit had the following: a couple of rooms, each of which had three beds and three dressers; a couple of quiet rooms, where "out-of-control" patients were put until they settled down; one pay phone; and one central bathroom, which consisted of two sinks, two stalls, two urinals, and a shower (and a bathtub?). I assume the female unit was similar. These two units were separated by a common area, called the dayroom, which had a television, a couple of couches, a few tables with chairs, and a refrigerator. The nurses' station was across from the dayroom.

Most of the days and evenings were spent in the dayroom, where patients stared mindlessly at the television or just into space. Privileges were very few. Occasionally, someone from occupational therapy would come to entertain us (e.g., drawing or bingo), or a doctor might allow a patient to go to the occupational-therapy room, but that was it.

Bournewood was different from any hospital I had been in before, except for Florida State. I would not call it bad, but it came closer to fitting the mold of the stereotypic mental institution than any of the other hospitals did–again with the exception of Florida State. (Actually, I shouldn't be too hard on Bournewood–it wasn't really that bad–just old.) I have already described the setting. There were also a number of strict rules. For instance, because some patients had violent or suicidal tendencies, no one was allowed to keep any personal belongings. Pocket combs, toothbrushes, toothpaste, shampoo, etc. were all kept locked. The staff, most of whom were friendly, brought meals to the dayroom. Utensils were counted before and after meals. There was little choice of food. You had what you were sent, occasionally having a few options. Many patients were heavy smokers and they had to be allotted cigarettes and get a match from the staff. My mother always did my laundry and made sure I had clean clothes. Other patients were not as lucky to have someone like my mom. Their laundry was gathered together and sent out.

Visiting hours were from six to eight, weeknights, and two to eight, weekends. As you can guess, my parents visited me every day. This provided me with an opportunity to get off the locked ward, which was on the second floor. Since there was no elevator and my dad could not come up to see me, I was allowed to go downstairs to visit (a staff member would always accompany me and remain close by). There was one week that my mom did not visit me–she had to be hospitalized for thyroid surgery. Fortunately, this surgery went very well, and the hospitalization was for only a few days. During this time, my father visited us both, despite the inconvenience and difficulty caused by the wheel-chair. My brother and he would visit my mother in one hospital, then come to see me in another. Was that dedication or what?

I entered Bournewood at 81 pounds. The first couple of weeks were uneventful. I refused to gain weight, though I did maintain. We were at an impasse. It was obvious that my staying at Bour-newood was pointless. This was not a hospital for food prob-lems, as you could probably gather from my description of the facility. Realizing this, Dr. Wiener arranged for me to be trans-ferred to the eating-disorders unit of Children's Hospital in Bos-ton. He was able to arrange this transfer thanks to the assistance of Dr. Nauss, who was affiliated with Children's. (Talk about a small world–Dr. Nauss and Dr. Wiener knew each other because Dr. Nauss had been the pediatrician for Dr. Wiener's children.) There was a waiting list, and so I had to spend another couple of weeks at Bournewood. I left on April 13, still weighing 81 pounds.

Chapter 14

Tricks at Children's Hospital

Children's Hospital was known for its eating-disorders unit, the Judge Baker Psychiatric Unit. I had been in therapy for anorexia for almost four years, but this was the first time I'd be in treatment at a place that specialized in food problems, with doctors trained to deal with this specific issue. To this day, my mom feels that Dr. P should have recommended a place like Children's for me. She believes that if he had done so—before my problems escalated—then things never would have gotten to the point they are at now.

The program at Children's, considered one of the best in the country, was very structured. It consisted of individual therapy, group therapy, occupational therapy, and a strict regimen concerning meals. Each patient was treated individually, based on his needs. I was one of a few anorexics. Although it was an eating-disorders unit, patients were there for other reasons also, some simply because they had difficulty getting along with their parents. At age nineteen, I was the oldest patient; all the others were adolescents.

One difference between Children's and all the other hospitals I had been in, or would later be in, was visiting hours. Visitors were allowed only on weekends and Tuesday nights (it may have been Wednesdays—I'm not sure). This was a change for me. Before, I had always seen my parents at least once a day.

The Tuesday-night visits, referred to as Family Night, followed a set schedule. During the day, we, the patients, prepared a meal for our parents. Parents arrived in the evening, and there would be a group session (including parents) of all the patients who had eating disorders. After this session, we had dinner and visited. Some of the patients, myself included, were on certain diets, and therefore, our dinners would be different from those given to our parents. My last memory of my father took place at one of these dinners. He asked me to get him a cup of ginger ale. I don't know why I specifically remember this, I just do. Maybe because it has to do with food, which was always an issue.

I said that each patient had his own food program. Personally, I was expected to gain 3 1/3 pounds per week. When I did not meet this requirement, I had to consume an eight-ounce, 250-calorie can of Ensure. (Ensure is a supplement drink, high in calories, protein, and other nutrients. There are many similar drinks on the market.) This, plus an increase of 250 calories per day.

I started out at 1,250 calories per day. The meals were carefully supervised. The staff was responsible for watching the patients and making sure that we had everything we were supposed to. For example, one evening, my dinner included a baked potato. A baked potato was something I frequently had when I was younger, before the food problems began. I was raised and taught to cut the potato in half, have the inside, and throw away the outer brown skin. That evening, I did this and was accused by the person watching me of trying to get away with not having my complete dinner. "That's stupid," I told her. "If I wanted to deceive anyone, I would not leave the skin out in the open. Besides, it's only a potato skin. What's the big deal? I left it because that's what I'm supposed to do. I'm not supposed to eat it. I have always thrown it away." She wouldn't listen to me, and I had to eat the potato skin.

No matter how closely a patient was watched, there were many ways to trick the staff. I was able to fool them as often as I felt like it. At home or in other hospitals, when I did not have what I was supposed to, I simply lied. No one was watching me or knew the difference. It was at Children's that I was supervised for the first time, and it was at Children's that I started using tricks.

Hiding food was the most common way of tricking the staff. I was not the only patient to do this, and I won't bother you with specific details. However, I will tell you about my all-time favorite trick, one that was exclusive to me. It was very original, and no one had any idea what I was doing.

All the tricks gave me a feeling of power. I would feel smarter than the staff–as if I were above them, getting back at them for watching me. (This, of course, was stupid; the only one I was hurting was myself.) This particular trick added to these feelings. I think the reason for this is that in the back of their minds, a lot of the staff would suspect some patients of hiding food, especially if we weren't gaining weight. However, in this case, no one had any idea what I was doing.

Each morning and evening, I received an eight-ounce carton of milk (the same kind that is given to children in elementary schools). One day, I got my hands on an unopened carton. I took it to the bathroom and with the tip of a pencil, made a tiny, unnoticeable hole in the bottom. I stood over a toilet, drained all the milk out of the carton, and put the carton in my coat pocket. When the next meal came up, it took just a moment to switch the empty carton with the one that had come up on the tray. After doing this, I deliberately made a show of opening the empty carton and pretending to drink the milk. I did this before anything else, so that the aides would not have an opportunity to discover that a switch had been made. They were totally oblivious to what had happened. As far as they were concerned, I had consumed my milk. Later, I would take the carton which I had removed from the tray, drain it, and repeat the whole process.

I did this trick for a couple of weeks, but was eventually caught when the staff searched my locker and found some empty cartons. Two milk cartons per day (150 calories each) may not seem like much, but they added up. When combined with other cutbacks, they made a difference, at least to me (to you, I'm sure it sounds stupid and foolish).

Because of all the cutbacks, I understandably did not gain any weight–I was having only about half of the calories I was supposed to consume. When I did not gain the expected weight, I had to have a can of Ensure. I decided to try the milk-carton trick with the Ensure can. This, however, was more difficult because the can was made of steel, not cardboard. By the time I finished making a hole, the can was rather bent out of shape, so I did this trick only once or twice.

I hesitate to write about these or any other tricks. I don't want another anorexic to read about and use them. After all, one or two ideas I had about deceiving workers came from other patients, which supports my belief that psychiatrists and psychiatric hospitals are pointless, if not detrimental. However, hopefully, more doctors, nurses, aides, and health workers will read this book, know what to look for, and be more careful.

Chapter 15

On Again, Off Again

Children's Hospital did help me. At first–before starting with the tricks–I made a good deal of progress. For the first time, my family and I believed that I was getting better. In the first few weeks that I was there, I followed the program, cooperated, and managed to gain about 10 or 11 pounds. Furthermore, I got along well with my therapist, Ms. F, who I called by her first name. Even though I was gaining weight, I did not feel fat–or at least not so fat that I couldn't accept the feelings. Being with other anorexics, my thoughts of competition, which had been present for the first time at Norwood Hospital (see the last paragraph of Chapter 4), were at their strongest, but I was able to tolerate them.

If you recall, I mentioned that I had stopped having lunch around the beginning of 1986 (Chapter 8). Well, at Children's, I even tried to eat lunch. This is what I mean when I tell you that I made progress there. To you, having lunch may seem trivial, but to me, it was a major step. I was still depressed, but as far as food was concerned, things were looking up.

This did not last. After the first couple of weeks, my weight stabilized. I was increased to 1,500 calories a day and continued to willingly comply with the program. My weight increased to 92 pounds, and I was "satisfied." However, when my weight once again stabilized, I was increased to 1,750 calories. This is when the trouble began. I started to feel fat and began with the tricks. Because I was not actually having the 1,750 calories, there was no change in my weight, and my calories were increased to 2,000.

This really bothered me. After all, I weighed 92 pounds—the most I had been since leaving St. Elizabeth's the previous December. It had taken a long time for me to accept this weight, but I had. "Give me time to adjust to the 92," I said. "What's the rush? I've been at such a low weight for so long, that another couple of weeks won't make a difference. Better that I gain at my own pace, slowly and voluntarily, than to force it on me, have me rebel, and ruin everything we've accomplished so far. Perhaps, given time, I'll be willing to accept a higher weight. But for now, 90 to 95 is my limit. Anything else will be too much, too soon."

I just didn't understand why everyone could not be satisfied with the 90 to 95; I was. However, I guess what I felt didn't matter. Everyone else knew what was best for me. I was told that the 2,000 calories and additional weight gain were requirements. The plan was for me to get up to 110 to 120 pounds. To me, this was unthinkable.

Using different tricks, I had been able to keep from going above 92 pounds for a little while. However, once my calories were increased to 2,000, I decided it was time for me to leave. For the couple of weeks preceding this, ever since my calories had been increased to 1,750, taking off had been on my mind. I knew that by keeping my weight stagnant, I was just postponing the inevitable. Furthermore, Ms. F told me that my weight gain would have to be completed at a different hospital. Children's Hospital allowed only a two-month stay, and reaching 110 to 120 pounds would require more than my remaining time. This would mean starting all over in a new setting with new doctors, new staff, and a new program. I felt overwhelmed. On May 24, I ran.

Chapter 16

A Letter Home

When I left Children's, I did not bother with the bus. I didn't think I had the time. When I had left Emerson, I knew no one would realize I was gone until the early evening, because I was not due back until the end of the day. However, in this case, I wasn't supposed to leave the hospital at all, and so I knew that I would soon be missed. I went to Logan Airport, took an express shuttle to La Guardia Airport in New York, flew to North Carolina, and then checked into a hotel. It was my intention to just lie on the bed in this hotel room and fast until I died.

How was I able to pay for a plane ticket and hotel room? Well, on April 30, on a pass home from the hospital, I withdrew some money from the bank (yes, they goofed again). I had been holding on to this money, hidden, for three and a half weeks.

Back home, there were newspaper articles about me and pleas for any information as to my whereabouts. (See Figures 16.1, 16.2, 16.3, and 16.4.) To this day, I don't know why, but seven days after leaving Children's, I was still alive. I called home and told my parents where I was (during the whole week, this was the only time I called them—imagine what they must have been going through). My mom flew to North Carolina and brought me home. (See Figure 16.5.) Yes, I agree with what you are now probably thinking—my parents did not deserve to get stuck with me; I did not deserve to be given such great parents; and yes, I am a pathetic human being.

Before leaving for La Guardia, I mailed a letter to my parents and brother that I had been writing for some time.

FIGURE 16.1

Parents fear for son who left hospital

A 19-year-old man suffering from anorexia nervosa and severe depression walked out of Children's Hospital Tuesday morning where he was being treated, and has not been seen since.

The parents of Michael Krasnow said they believe their son, who is 5 feet 10 inches tall and weighs only 90 pounds, has run away.

Hospital officials fear Krasnow will starve himself to death if not found soon.

Krasnow, who is from Framingham, was wearing a tan winter coat, off-white pants and Nike sneakers when he left the hospital. He has brown hair and is extremely thin.

"They think he's not going to eat," said Phil Lotane, a hospital spokesman. "He wants to starve himself to death, and, obviously, at 90 pounds he doesn't have far to go."

Krasnow's father, Jerry, said that shortly after his son left the hospital, he emptied his bank account. Jerry Krasnow said that judging from notes written by his son, he may have taken a plane or bus westward, or perhaps to Florida.

"He may have gone to Houston or California just for a complete change. He has enough money to travel anywhere."

Krasnow was on earned free time when he left the hospital at about 9:30 a.m., but was not supposed to leave the building. When he did not return by 11, authorities were notified, Lotane said.

Police and airline officials have been notified and a nationwide all points bulletin has been released, Jerry Krasnow said.

—AMY CALLAHAN

Article by Amy Callahan from *The Boston Globe*, May 25, 1988. (Reprinted courtesy of *The Boston Globe*.)

FIGURE 16.2

'Troubled' teen flees hospital

By NICK TATE

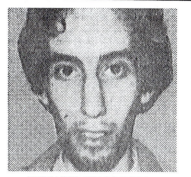

MICHAEL KRASNOW
Could die without treatment

A TROUBLED teen-age anorexic, whose father fears may have a "death wish," fled a Hub hospital psychiatric ward this week, sparking a massive search yesterday to find him before he dies.

Michael Krasnow, a 19-year-old Framingham youth suffering from anorexia nervosa, slipped past medical staff at the Judge Baker Guidance Center of Children's Hospital Monday, triggering frantic moves by police and family members to track him down.

Krasnow, who at 5-foot-10 weighs only 90 pounds, was undergoing counseling and treatment at the ward for the psychiatric eating disorder and clinical depression when he escaped, hospital spokesman Phil Lotane said.

"From a medical standpoint he's going to die if he's not found soon," Lotane said. "He may be trying to starve himself to death; that's why we're so fearful."

Jerry Krasnow, the teen's father, explained that the former honors student has had a five-year history of psychological problems—including depression, anorexia and obsessive-compulsive behavior—that kept him in and out of hospitals.

Family members said Krasnow, who at 19 is his own guardian, withdrew his savings from a bank account shortly after leaving the hospital—an indication he may have left the area.

Krasnow, of 14 Central St., has brown eyes and hair and was wearing a khaki jacket and white pants when last seen.

Article by Nick Tate from the *Boston Herald*, May 25, 1988. (Reprinted by permission of the *Boston Herald*.)

FIGURE 16.3

Desperate plea for missing teen

THE ANGUISHED father of a missing anorexic teen, who fled the psychiatric ward of a Boston hospital last week, issued a new appeal yesterday that his son be found before it's too late.

Jerry Krasnow, whose 19-year-old son, Michael, escaped from a Children's Hospital ward last, said the risk his emaciated son will die of starvation grows every day he remains missing.

"He can't afford to lose more weight. They told me at the hospital he's a candidate for sudden death."

Michael is 5-foot-10, with brown hair and eyes and was wearing a khaki jacket and off-white pants when last seen.

Anyone with information that could lead to his whereabouts is asked to call Boston police, who are investigating the case.

Article from the *Boston Herald*, May 30, 1988. (Reprinted by permission of the *Boston Herald*.)

FIGURE 16.4

Framingham teen missing from Boston hospital

Parents fear for anorexic son

By the News Staff

FRAMINGHAM – Nineteen-year-old Michael Krasnow, 5-foot, 10-inches and 90 pounds, walked out of Children's Hospital last Tuesday and hasn't been seen or heard from since.

The Framingham teen-ager suffers from anorexia nervosa and depression, and because of his illness he starves himself to the point of medical emergency. If he doesn't get medical and psychiatric help, Michael's parents and hospital officials fear he will die. And if he is not found soon, he won't get the help he needs.

"If he were healthy, we wouldn't be worried. We're not doting parents, we're not parents who are afraid to cut the strings," said Jerry Krasnow from his Temple Street home. "We're worried because he's not well, because of his illness."

Michael had been at Children's Hospital since April 13 and had permission to leave his floor when he left last Tuesday and failed to return.

Since his freshman year at Framingham North, Michael has been depressed and obsessive, with anorexia nervosa, a life-threatening psychiatric disorder that gives people a false body image. Sufferers, most of whom are teen-age girls, believe they are fat and literally starve themselves in a quest to be thin and exercise control over their bodies.

Krasnow disappeared last November, walking away from the Babson College

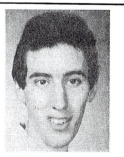

Michael Krasnow

campus. Krasnow was found in Orlando, Fla., several days later, after a search that included advertisements in local and Boston newspapers.

Since April 13, Michael had gained about 10 pounds from his all-time low of 80, according to his parents, "but had not turned the corner."

Michael's parents believe their son may have run away because of his planned discharge from Children's. They believe he may have been panicky about having to start over again with new therapists.

Michael was never overweight. At Framingham North he was a member of the freshman track and basketball teams, and "had a terrific build like an athlete," according to Jerry Krasnow.

But once he became anorexic, Michael's weight dropped below 100 pounds and has never gone back up. He is not physically strong, and the lack of food has affected his thinking. Doctors say he can not live much longer without eating.

Michael was last seen wearing off-white jeans, Nike sneakers, a dress shirt and a beige down jacket that hung to just above his knees. His mother said Michael is likely wearing the winter jacket even in hot, sunny weather.

Jerry and Gail Krasnow urge anyone who thinks they may have seen their son to call Boston police.

From the *Middlesex News*, May 28, 1988. (Reprinted by permission of the *Middlesex News*, Framingham, Massachusetts.)

FIGURE 16.5

Runaway teen found in North Carolina

FRAMINGHAM — A local run-away teen-ager suffering from anorexia nervosa has been found in a North Carolina motel, according to his parents.

FRAMINGHAM

Jerry Krasnow of Temple Street said his 19-year-old son, Michael, is being brought back home by his mother, who flew to North Carolina to find the teen.

From the *Middlesex News* (no date). (Reprinted by permission of the *Middlesex News*, Framingham, Massachusetts.)

Dear Mom, Dad, and Neil,
Running away has been in the back of my mind for some time now. Up to this point, I've successfully been able to fight the urge (the one thing that has kept me going is my love for you). Children's has an excellent program (this is by far the best hospital for anorexics), and I know that I've made progress here; it's too bad that I couldn't stick it out. If I am caught and have my choice of hospitals, I'd hope that Children's would give me a second chance (I've made more progress here than at all the other hospitals combined). I've found that I can talk with Ms. F and the staff, but I still feel fat. This just further verifies that I'm a loser and a failure.

Please, never forget that *I love you.* You're the greatest family a person could ask for. I don't deserve to have you as a family, and it's a shame that you got stuck with me.

It's too bad that no one can accept me at my present weight. As I've told you many times before, I'm willing to maintain, but I would rather die than gain a pound (I could live with a 5- to 10-pound weight gain, but not 20 to 30 pounds).

I have enclosed my new bankbook. If I had taken money out of my account, you would have noticed. Therefore, I reported my bankbook as being lost and got a new one. This enabled me to withdraw money without your knowing. The old bankbook in my dresser drawer is now no good.

Let me remind you one last time: I love all three of you and pray that you can be happy.

Love,
Michael

* * *

This letter was written on May 1. It is now May 13. For two weeks, I've been successfully fighting the urge to run. Today, I found that my calories are increased to 2,000; this discovery has pushed me over the edge, and I've given in to my urges. My running today was not planned. I've been fighting the urges day by day. I learned of the increase and just panicked.

I do not want to die. I want to live, but I feel as though I'm being backed into a wall. If I was allowed to maintain my weight at 90 to 95, then I'd continue living, but everyone wants me to gain weight. I do not want to die, but right now, I don't feel I have a choice.

Maybe I won't kill myself. I'll just take the bus to Florida, find a job and a place to live, and start my life over again. I'll prove to you and everyone else that I can make it on my own. My life has been screwed up for the past few years, and I just want a chance to start over.

Since April 30, I have fought and fought with myself and my urges; I guess I just can't do it anymore.

* * *

Mom and Dad, it's May 23, and Ms. F just told me that I'll have to go to another hospital for a month or so. This means that I will not be coming home for a while. All I want is for you to be happy, but I cannot fight these feelings anymore. Please, remember I love you. The only thing that was keeping me going was saying to myself, "Michael, just wait until June 3, and then you can be home." Now that I am going to another hospital, there is nothing to keep me going.

Learning that I have to go to another hospital instead of home is "the straw that broke the camel's back." It is the thing that has made me give in to my urges. I just don't have the motivation to go to another hospital and start all over with someone new.

It's a shame that this is happening because I feel I've made such a huge amount of progress here. Right now, I'm scared and confused. Mom and Dad, you can ask any nurse or doctor at Children's Hospital. Everyone knows that I've been keeping myself alive for one reason and one reason only. That reason is my love for you. The best parents in the world got stuck with a loser for a son.

Believe it or not, I'm 92 pounds, but I do not feel obese. I could live with maintaining this weight. However, between now and June 3, they want me to gain at least five more pounds. Why can't anyone be satisfied with 92? I would be quite comfortable at 92. Instead of being satisfied with my progress, the hospital is increasing my calories and pushing me over the edge.

I know I failed once before trying to maintain a weight of 90 to 95, but I know that I could do it if I was given a second chance (this is part of what I mean when I say that I've made progress).

Chapter 17

I Gain a Guardian
and Lose a Father

Upon being brought back from North Carolina, I was admitted to Newton-Wellesley Hospital in Newton, Massachusetts. It was June 1. I had fasted for eight days (the last time I had eaten was 7:50 a.m. on Tuesday, May 24) and still refused to have anything. I was immediately hooked up to an IV. As I have frequently mentioned, the last time I had a drink of water was February 1985. Therefore, a fast for me is literally a fast. Understandably, my weight was down to 74 pounds. Most of this was fluid loss, and when the IV started, this alone helped my weight. At 5:15 p.m., on Thursday, June 2, I had eight ounces of juice and a can of Ensure. In a span of 225 hours and 25 minutes, all that I had accomplished at Children's Hospital was ruined.

Once I started eating at Newton-Wellesley, even though it was very minimal, my weight went up to 80 pounds. It would remain there during my entire stay at Newton-Wellesley, which would be approximately one month. Every day was the same. In the morning, I had a bagel with cream cheese and eight ounces of pineapple juice; in the evening, I had a tuna fish or turkey sandwich (with mayonnaise) and eight ounces of apple juice.

In addition to working out of Bournewood, Dr. Wiener was affiliated with Newton-Wellesley, and he was once again my doctor. On June 20, Dr. Wiener wrote a deposition to the probate court in Dedham, Massachusetts, and requested that my mother be granted temporary guardianship over me. I decided that it would be pointless to fight the guardianship, and since I didn't really care, I voluntarily consented to it.

This temporary guardianship gave my mother power over all my money (this was immaterial–I had taken money out of the bank before, even though I wasn't supposed to), as well as the right to authorize my being given surgery, medications, tube feedings, and IV fluids.

Basically, she was given the right to consent to my receiving any medication or other treatment that might help get me better, or in an emergency, save my life. As a special power, she was given the right to authorize electroshock therapy (ECT).

The temporary guardianship was granted at the end of June. At the same time, I voluntarily went back to Bournewood and agreed to ECT.

I returned to Bournewood on June 30–still 80 pounds–and immediately started a series of thirteen ECT treatments. More about that later. First, I would like to pay tribute to my father, one of the two greatest people who ever lived (the other one, of course, is my mother).

As you know, my father suffered from ALS. On July 7, seven days after my admittance to Bournewood, my father passed away. Gerald Krasnow was special. Most of my memories, those of times before the anorexia, are of things I did with my parents.

My father's love and devotion for his family–me in particular– were demonstrated by how he treated me after the anorexia started. He was willing to pursue anything that might help me. Time, money, etc.–there were no obstacles. He was always there for me, always hopeful. His greatest wish was for me to get better.

I've told you how great my dad was, so I'm going to hate myself for saying this, but I don't miss him. I don't even think about him that much. I know I'm an ungrateful, good-for-nothing jerk, who never deserved such a great father, but it's the truth. I also know it's because of the depression. This is no excuse, but I just don't care about anyone or anything.

Chapter 18

Effects of ECT

ECT is most commonly used to help those who suffer from severe depression, usually as a last resort when psychotherapy, medication, etc., have proven unsuccessful. One of the possible side effects of ECT is memory loss, and this was the most prevalent result of my treatment. Therefore, much of what I write about this period comes from what I have been told by others or from notes I kept during this time. To the best of my knowledge, everything is accurate, but I cannot guarantee it.

The ECT was done two or three times per week. The evening before a treatment, I was not supposed to have anything to eat after dinner. Since I had only breakfast and dinner, this did not faze me, but I think it was rather ironic. I mean, I wasn't willing to eat, but what if I had been? If I was in the hospital to gain weight, and wanted something to eat, would I have been told that I couldn't?

First thing in the morning, I would be taken to the ECT room. While I lay on a table, the nurse used glue to stick white patches all over my body; these patches were attached to wires. I was then given a shot of an anesthetic, which instantly put me to sleep. Next thing I knew, I would wake up a few hours later—about ten or eleven o'clock. After waking up, it would be okay to eat, and of course in my case, I was immediately rushed to have the breakfast I had missed.

Undoubtedly, the worst thing about this time is my inability to remember my dad's last days. On the day of my father's death, my uncle picked me up at Bournewood and took me to see him. My dad was also in a hospital. Imagine, every day my mother would go to one hospital to visit him, and then to another hospital to see me.

From what my mom tells me, I requested to have some time alone with my dad. It's a shame that I do not recall anything of these final moments. I have no idea what I said to him. According to my mother, I told my dad, "Everything's okay. I'm having ECT and feel much better. I'm getting stronger each day. Everything's great." But I just don't remember.

Actually, as I sit here writing this and checking dates, it has just occurred to me that my father died about one and a half months after I ran from Children's. Did the stress and worry of my running speed up his deterioration and bring about his death that much quicker?

The ECT did help the depression a little bit; I was also able to gain 8 pounds. I was discharged from Bournewood on July 29, weighing 88 pounds. The plan was for me to see Dr. Wiener two times a week on an outpatient basis. Unfortunately, the lessening of depression lasted only a couple of months, and I was soon as depressed as ever. In Dr. Wiener's office on August 9, I voluntarily consented to the temporary guardianship being converted to a permanent one. I knew my mom would do only what was best for me (at least, what she thought was best), and besides, I just didn't care.

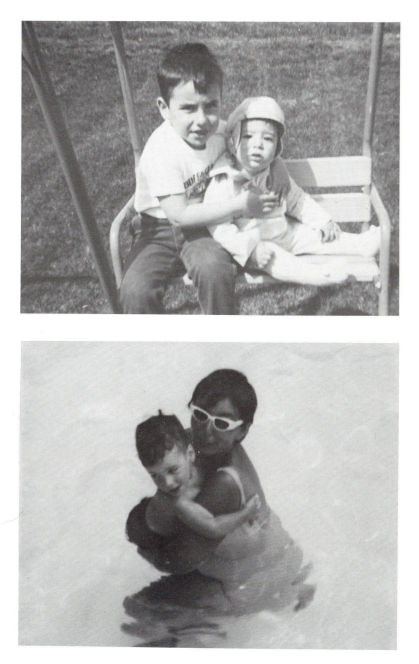

PHOTO 1 (top): Me and Neil, 1970 (Age 1). PHOTO 2 (bottom): With Mom, 1971 (Age 2).

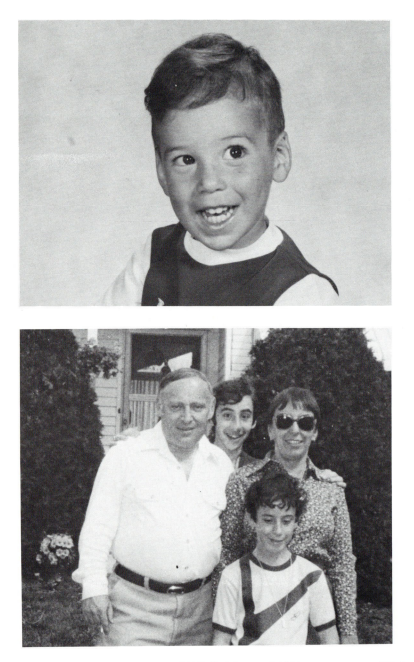

PHOTO 3 (top): Me, 1973 (Age 4). PHOTO 4 (bottom): With my parents and Neil, 1976? (Age 7).

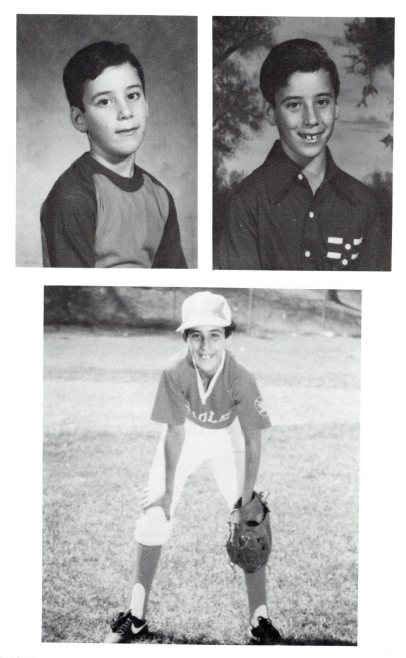

PHOTO 5 (top, left): Grade 2, 1977 (Age 8). PHOTO 6 (top, right): Grade 4, 1979 (Age 10). PHOTO 7 (bottom): Little League baseball, Summer 1981 (Age 12).

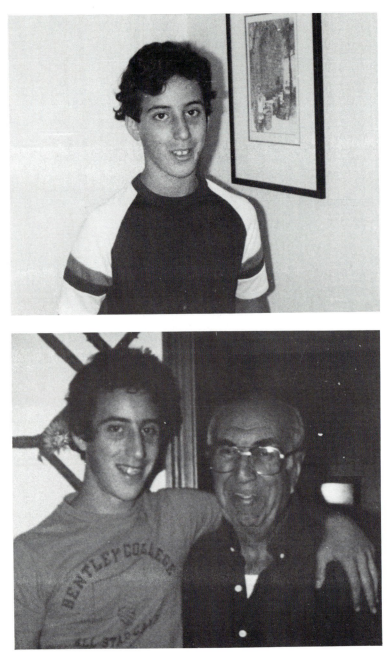

PHOTO 8 (top): 1982 (Age 13). PHOTO 9 (bottom): With my grandfather, 1983 (Age 14).

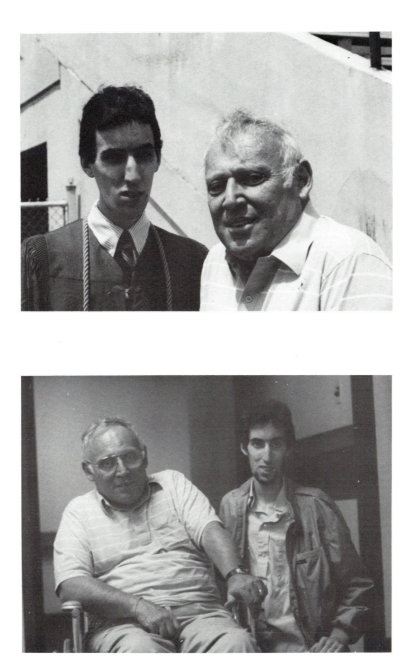

PHOTO 10 (top): High school graduation with my dad, June 1987 (Age 18).
PHOTO 11 (bottom): Me and Dad (one month before he died), June 1988 (Age 19).

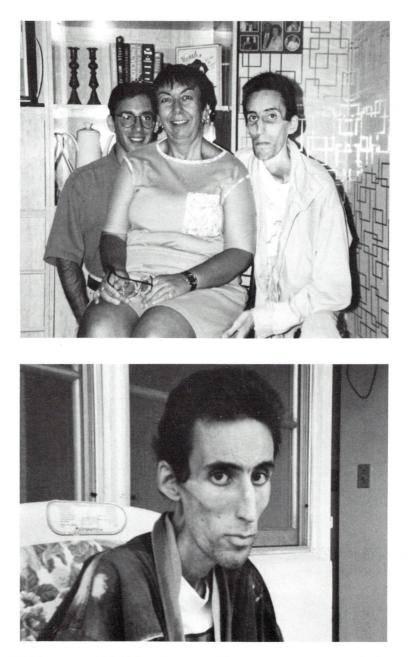

PHOTO 12 (top): With Neil and my mom, October 1995 (Age 26). PHOTO 13 (bottom): Me, October 1995 (Age 26).

Chapter 19

Back Home–Again

After I returned home, my day-to-day life fell back into the same pattern it had followed for the past few years. I went back to the library. Everyone there had been extremely nice. They sent me get-well cards in the hospital and sympathy cards when my dad passed away. Can you believe that they would take me back again? Just goes to show how kind, caring, and open-minded some people are. Since I could get only a small number of hours there, I took a second part-time job, working in the library of the Harvard University Primate Research Center.

At first, things were uneventful. But of course, as you can guess, since I am such a failure, I started to lose weight. On April 3, 1989, I left my two part-time jobs in favor of one full-time job. I was in charge of a small library in a research-consulting firm. This was your typical, nine-to-five job. Still, albeit slowly, I lost weight.

At the end of June, I was scheduled for my semiannual checkup with Dr. Nauss. Although Dr. Nauss was a pediatrician, and I was twenty years old, I continued to see him. He had been my doctor for almost my entire life, knew all about me, and more important, I thought he cared. At this time, I weighed only 74 pounds. Yes, 74. Why had no one done anything? Well, my mother and Dr. Wiener didn't know that I was losing weight. I'm sure they suspected, but I lied. (Dr. Wiener did not weigh me; he would ask about my weight, and I'd say that everything was the same.) Besides, even though I had lost fourteen pounds since leaving Bournewood, a weight loss is not as noticeable when it takes place slowly. This was especially true in my mother's case, because she saw me every day.

I knew that once my appointment with Dr. Nauss revealed my weight loss, I would be hospitalized. A few days before this appointment, my mother wanted to weigh me on our scale at home. I "tricked" her by attaching two seven-and-a-half-pound ankle weights to myself. I wasn't sure what I was going to do about my upcoming appointment with Dr. Nauss. As usual, I was thinking of taking off. To this day, I can't understand why I could not be allowed to stay at 74 pounds. True, that number is unthinkable in medical fields. However, every individual is different. If I was able to work forty hours a week and function at 74 pounds, then I should have been left alone. It was—and still is—my life.

Anyway, what I would or would not have done is a moot point. On June 20, the day my mother weighed me, I went to work. As it turned out, I didn't completely fool my mom. I had lost 14 pounds; even though the scale had read 89, she knew by looking at me that this just couldn't be true. After I left for work, she searched my room and found the ankle weights. A few hours later, she walked into where I was working and told me that the police were waiting outside in order to take me to the hospital. Well, I had no choice, so I went.

Chapter 20

The Last Hospital Story

At this point, you're probably getting tired of hearing the same old story about the hospital. Well, this will be the last one.

The police took me to Newton-Wellesley Hospital, where I was admitted to the psychiatric unit. Here, I continued with Dr. Wiener, and also met Dr. Theodore Spielberg, the third of the three "good" doctors I mentioned earlier. Actually, we had met the previous year, during my first stay at Bournewood, but only briefly.

Dr. Spielberg went out of his way to help me. How many doctors do you know who will bring books, comic books, games, etc., to their patients (and pay for these with their own money)? He really cared. Dr. Spielberg did not want just to do his job and send me home. He wanted to help me to enjoy life and not simply exist. (Note to Drs. Nauss, Wiener, and Spielberg: If you read this book, and I'm sure you will since I intend to send each of you a copy, I mean everything I've said—I really think you guys cared about me—thank you.)

Between June 20 and June 28, there was a lot of confusion. I kept a few notes during this time, but I'm still not sure exactly what happened. What I do know is that on June 28, I weighed 69 1/4 pounds. I was transferred to the medical floor in order to be force-fed. Force-feeding is done through tubes placed in the nose. I ripped these tubes out of my nose. On June 30, I was down to 67 3/4 pounds. That afternoon, Dr. Spielberg and I came to an agreement.

Dr. Spielberg was willing to work with me. He said I'd have to gain weight—maintaining would be no good—but listened when I told him that for this to happen, it would need to be done slowly. You see, Dr. Spielberg did not try to be a magician and "make" me better. I'm sure he would have liked to, but he knew that it wouldn't happen. Unlike many doctors, he had some intelligence; he knew we had to work together.

According to our agreement, I was to have 800 calories per day, plus one 240-calorie can of Sustacal (similar to Ensure)—a total of 1,040 calories. If at any time my weight dropped, I would increase my calories by 250.

On July 2, my weight was 67 pounds, which meant I had to increase 250 calories. I was willing to do this. However, Dr. V, who was covering for the vacationing Dr. Spielberg, now entered the picture.

I "blame" Dr. V for all the problems that would happen over the next five months. Now, I know it was absolutely, 100 percent, my own fault and no one else's. I was in control of my actions and had the ability to change what I was doing, eat something, etc., etc. However, if Dr. V had not appeared, I would have voluntarily eaten the agreed-upon 1,290 calories. Maybe all of what I am about to tell you would have happened anyway, but I don't think so.

When Dr. V came on his rounds that day, I explained the contract to him, as well as my plans to cooperate and follow it. "I have an agreement with Dr. Spielberg," I told him. "Since my weight went down, I'm supposed to increase my calories by 250, and I'll do that."

Dr. V replied that the contract was null and void—I was going to be force-fed. Now tell me, what right did he have to break the agreement? As I said, his interference ruined everything.

The tube feedings started at about 6:30 p.m. on July 2. I refused to voluntarily swallow the tubes (the tubes go through the nose and down to the stomach, but in order for them to be placed correctly, the patient needs to swallow), so the doctor had to force them down me. Nine times he pushed them in and yanked them out. I started to cough up blood. Later, the nurse would tell me, "It was so gross, that I had to turn away."

After finally getting the tubes in place, the doctor decided to tie my wrists, so that I couldn't pull out the tubes. I was fed 12 1/2 calories per hour. Does this make sense to you? At this rate, I would have 300 calories per day, which was a lot less than I was willing to have voluntarily. The 12 1/2 calories would eventually be increased, but still . . .

Even though my wrists were tied to the bed, I managed to pull out the tubes at about 2:30 a.m. (I intentionally waited until this hour, figuring that it would be less likely for a doctor to be available to replace them.) In other words, I received 100 calories from the tubes. If Dr. V had not interfered, I would have voluntarily eaten 1,290 calories.

On July 3, I weighed only 66 1/4 pounds. Dr. V called and said, "The tubes did not work out, so just have 1,000 calories today."

"This guy's an idiot," I told my mom. "Yesterday, 1,290 calories was not okay, but today, 1,000 calories is. Well, forget it. Why should I do what he says, and then have Dr. Wiener or someone else come by and change everything? With so many different doctors telling me so many different things, it just leads to confusion. I have two doctors–Dr. Wiener and Dr. Spielberg– and I'm not doing anything until the three of us sit down together and come to an understanding. Until then, I'm just going to fast. Let them put the tubes down my nose. I don't care. I'll just rip them out again. I'm not doing anything until Dr. Spielberg returns. Hopefully, I'll die before he gets back."

Dr. Spielberg was not scheduled to return until July 10. From July 3 until July 10, things became rather hectic. Throughout this week, feeding tubes were placed in my nose on thirteen separate occasions, and I yanked them out on thirteen separate occasions. I did this, despite being assigned a "sitter," whose job was to do nothing except watch me and make sure that I didn't pull out the tubes.

How, then, was I able to free myself of them? Easy–the sitters just fell asleep. My wrists were tied to the bed, but I still, somehow, managed to take out the tubes.

On July 5, I had a respiratory arrest, caused by hypoglycemia (low blood sugar), and needed to be transferred to the Intensive

Care Unit overnight. I continued to have attacks of hypoglycemia, and on July 8, had another respiratory arrest and needed to be revived.

When I had this respiratory arrest, my mother was on the phone with Dr. Wiener. If my uncle and a nurse had not been in the room at the time, I probably would have died. I recall that while I was "out," I told myself, "Wait twenty-four hours to die. Jason's [my cousin] planning to drive a couple of hours to visit you tomorrow, and you haven't had a chance to say good-bye to him."

Jason and I were very close as children. I sometimes describe him as having been "more like a brother than a cousin." As a teenager, he was a bit mischievous. However, he turned himself around and eventually graduated college, got his master's degree, and was named one of the Outstanding Young Men of America. He has a lot to be proud of and is on his way to being very successful.

Anyway, after the second respiratory arrest, there were more complications. On July 7, the day before the second arrest, because the tube feedings were ineffective, I had received a TPN (total parenteral nutrition). This is similar to tube feedings, but instead of sticking them through the nose, the tubes are sewn into the neck. As a result of the TPN, I suffered a collapsed (punctured) lung. This required sewing a tube into my chest in order to reinflate the lung.

On July 10, Dr. Spielberg returned. Although my fasting continued, I was getting some nutrition from the TPN. However, I was in no condition to start bargaining with him about gaining weight. The hypoglycemic attacks continued, and I spent each day going into and out of consciousness. I had severe anemia and needed blood transfusions. To prevent my pulling out the TPN, casts had been put on both my arms–in addition to my wrists still being tied down. I was pretty much immobile. I spent all day and evening lying in bed, covered with blankets because of hypothermia. Tubes were sewn into my neck and chest. The nurses had to turn me over every few hours to prevent my getting bed sores. I could not wash myself and needed to be bathed by the staff.

Getting to the bathroom was out of the question, so I needed to use a bedpan.

On July 14, it was discovered that I had severe bone-marrow failure, a result of malnutrition. My bones had been feeding off themselves–almost self-cannibalizing. I was treated for this with anabolic steroids by a Dr. O. One meeting that I had with Dr. O stands out in my mind. He wanted me to accept a shot for some reason–I don't remember exactly why. "If you do not take this shot, I am not going to treat you," he told me.

"Fine," I replied. "I don't care."

Dr. O did treat me. He later said that he should not have given me the ultimatum, and explained that most of his patients were terminally ill and would do anything to get better; he had no experience with someone who wanted to die.

On July 20, there was discussion about an operation. The idea was for me to receive a feeding gastrostomy. This is similar to a TPN, except the tubes are sewn into the stomach. The possibility was temporarily put on hold because on July 23, I received an infection, caused by the chest tube. My temperature went to 104 degrees, and I needed to receive antibiotics. Since I was still fasting and would not swallow anything, all medication had to be given to me as a shot or be administered anally. While this was going on, all my visitors–even the doctors and my mother–had to wear a surgical mask in order not to breathe any germs on me.

Around the end of July, the infection was gone. My bone marrow and collapsed lung were okay. I was no longer falling into unconsciousness and did not require any more blood transfusions. Talk of the operation resumed, and at this point–I don't know why–I agreed to start eating.

Once I began eating, the TPN was removed, and things settled down for a little while. Dr. Wiener and Dr. Spielberg continued to see me every day, and I received visits from a number of other people (these people had been visiting me since I had been hospitalized at the end of June). Of course, my mother came every day–she had even slept at the hospital when I was really bad. Other visitors included my uncle and his wife (who gave me a haircut), Jason, my Grandma Minnie, and David (another cousin). All of them visited me, even though they had to drive a couple of hours in order to get to the hospital. I told them not to waste their time coming—"I'm not worth it," I said—but they did. I also received visits from various friends of my mother's and the rabbi from my temple.

The one person whom I did not see was my brother, who was away from home. He was going to come visit me, but I said to my mom, "Don't tell Neil about all this [how bad I am and that I almost died]. I am such a jerk. I don't want him to leave his job to come see me. I've been enough of a problem, as it is, to so many people. I don't want to screw up his life."

On August 9, my weight was 69 3/4 pounds. Nobody in the hospital knew what to do with me. Everything had been tried—nothing had worked. The doctors met with my mother to discuss my receiving a second series of ECT treatments. Because of my condition, she was scared to give permission. However, the doctors convinced her that I'd die if not given the ECT, and so she signed the authorization slips.

The ECT began in the middle of August. Again, I do not remember anything of these treatments. All I recall is one "confrontation." There is not much point in my writing about this—it's not important—but I will, because it offers an excellent example of one of my most dominant traits—the need to feel in control.

One morning, a nurse sat down to watch me have my breakfast. "I want to make sure you have everything," she said.

"I'm not going to have you treat me like a baby, whose mother watches over him," I replied. "If you want to sit there, fine. But I'm not going to have anything while you're sitting there, staring at me."

She got up and left. To you, this seems stupid, but it was the type of thing which made me feel that I was the boss—"all-powerful" and in control.

I received twelve ECT treatments. However, they were uneventful. On October 12, weighing 71 1/2 pounds, I was transferred to Bournewood Hospital. I'm not really sure why. Supposedly, Dr. Wiener thought that while I was at Bournewood, he could convince me to check myself into a hospital with a specialized eating-disorders program.

I was at Bournewood for only one and a half weeks, and nothing happened there. I spent the entire time on the locked unit. I maintained my weight, but made no attempt to gain; I just sat in the dayroom and stared into space.

The hospital administrator believed I was wasting everyone's time (and I was), and she played a major role in my being discharged from Bournewood. She admitted that my being there worried her; she felt the hospital was taking a risk. Bournewood was a psychiatric facility, not a medical one, and wasn't equipped to deal with a medical emergency. On October 23, I was transferred back to Newton-Wellesley.

On November 9, I met Dr. M, a hypnotherapist. Because of difficulty concentrating, I could not be hypnotized. However, I continued to see Dr. M as a "regular" psychologist.

To make a long story short (actually, all I'm doing is bringing a long story to an end), I needed to reach 80 pounds in order to be allowed to go home. I don't know exactly when or why I decided to gain the weight, but I eventually did. On December 2, after about five and a half months in the hospital, I reached 80 pounds and was discharged.

Chapter 21

On My Own

Upon my release from Newton-Wellesley, everyone's main concern, of course, was that I would maintain my weight. Dr. Wiener and Dr. M wanted to continue seeing me, and I met with each of them once a week. I don't know why. I didn't care one bit about seeing them and got nothing out of the meetings. However, it made my mother feel better, and since it didn't matter to me, I complied and went.

In addition, I had weekly appointments with Dr. Spielberg, who kept tabs on my weight, which had to stay at 80 pounds. My mother also periodically checked my weight on the scale in our home.

Aside from my doctor appointments, I more or less did not get out of the house. Occasionally, as if I were a puppy dog, I'd tag along with my mother when she went to the mall, but that was it. I woke up in the morning, had my breakfast, sat down in a chair, and stared at the wall all day, sometimes turning on the TV. In the evening, I had my dinner and then vegetated some more. What kind of life was this? I had no desire to do anything; I simply wanted to die. I wasn't going to run again—I just didn't feel like it or have the motivation. Therefore, I decided to wait for an opportunity.

This opportunity came in the doctor's office, when my mother mentioned wanting to go to Florida to visit her mother. I saw my chance and jumped. I gave long speeches about how I was maintaining my weight, and emphasized other reasons why she should go. "I've been maintaining," I said to my mother and doctor (I do not recall whether it was Dr. Wiener or Dr. M).

"Mom, you deserve a vacation. Besides, you can't expect to hover over me all my life. Sooner or later, you won't be available and will have to leave me by myself."

Of course, you can probably guess what was going through my mind all this time. I would fast again–it would be ideal for me. I could die right at home–in my own bed–no need to run.

Supposedly, my condition could not get any worse than it had been at Newton-Wellesley (this had been the low point of my anorexia). Therefore, what I am about to tell you is almost anti-climactic.

The doctors agreed that my mother deserved a vacation, and she finally decided to take one. She left for Florida in January 1990, a little more than one month after my return from the hospital.

In our last meeting before my mom's departure, Dr. M said that he felt it was important for me to see him while my mother was gone. "That's stupid," I said. "I don't care about seeing you. I don't get anything out of our appointments. As far as I'm concerned, they're a waste of time and money. What's the big deal if I don't see you for a couple of weeks? Is the world going to come to an end?"

Dr. M still felt it was important, and said I could take a taxi to see him. "If you really want me to come that badly," I told him, "then fine, I'll come–if you're willing to pay for the cab." This shut him up, which goes to show you how "important" it was.

My mother's vacation was scheduled for four weeks, but I was by myself for only two of these. My brother, who had returned from his job, was living at home, and during the first two weeks my mother was gone, he took me to my doctor appointments. When Neil left to join my mother in Florida, I was by myself, and my fast began.

Throughout this book, I have repeated many times that I have not had a sip of water since February 1985. Therefore, when I speak of a fast, I mean a complete fast. I went one week with absolutely nothing entering my body. I have no idea why I am still alive. I mean, perfectly healthy people are supposed to be able to go only a short period without food or water. Here I was, a skeleton to begin with, and after a week of fasting, I was still alive.

During this fast (and the entire time she was gone), I spoke to my mother every day. "Everything's fine," I kept reassuring her.

Each time I've told you about my fasting, I've said that I don't know why I eventually "confessed" to what I was doing. This is again the case. After one week, I admitted what I was doing. Of course, my mother cried. Of course, I hated myself for being such a loser, a jerk, an idiot, a pathetic human being, and a complete waste. It was late in the afternoon. My mother said she was coming home on the first flight. I promised her that before going to bed, I would have a cup of juice, which I did, thus ending my fast. My mom returned late that evening, sometime after midnight. Her friends were kind enough to pick her up at the airport, even at that late hour.

In the morning, January 29, I had some juice and toast and was immediately taken to see Dr. Spielberg. My weight had gone from 80 pounds down to 68, and Dr. Spielberg wanted to hospitalize me. "That will do more harm than good," I told him. "I'm willing to get my weight back up. After all, I voluntarily told my mom what I was doing and have started eating. If you put me in the hospital, I'll fast. You can order the feeding tubes, but by the time that they get stuck in me, I'll probably be dead. And if I'm not, then we'll just end up with a repeat of what happened last time."

I guess Dr. Spielberg saw the futility of hospitalizing me. He agreed to let me stay out of the hospital and put the weight back on at my own pace. I think this was a noteworthy move on the part of Dr. Spielberg. For the first time in the entire course of my anorexia, I was told that I could get my weight back up in my own way. I could be wrong, but I believe that if I had been told this X number of years ago (e.g., at Children's Hospital–Chapters 14 and 15), much of what happened never would have. I did not feel that I was being bossed around or losing control. No one was saying, "You have to gain such and such a number of pounds in such and such an amount of time–or else." Dr. Spielberg was not trying to run my life and tell me what to do. He had brains enough to know that doing so would be pointless–and he was right.

Left to my own devices, I got my weight up from 68 to 75 pounds. I was supposed to go up to 80, but decided not to. Dr. Spielberg hinted at hospitalization to get me back to the 80, but I don't think he ever seriously considered it. He knew that if he hospitalized me, I would fast. It would be better for me to voluntarily maintain my weight at 75 pounds, which I did on 1,000 calories a day.

For the next nine or ten months, things remained the same. I continued with my weekly visits to Dr. Wiener, Dr. M, and Dr. Spielberg. Otherwise, I did very little. I tried reading, but although I was able to do some, I still had trouble concentrating. I sold my comic book collection, and occasionally looked for work.

Around December, my uncle visited us from Florida. He owned an insurance agency and mentioned that he would always have a job for me. One thing led to another. In February 1991, I moved to Hollywood, Florida, got my own studio apartment, and started working full-time for my uncle. My mother remained in Massachusetts.

Yes, you read it right. After all that had happened, why would I be allowed to live by myself? I can't really say. Probably, my mother and the doctors realized that nothing would be accomplished by my remaining at home. They had tried everything. Perhaps they thought that my being on my own would be good for me, maybe a stimulant.

I think being on my own has been good for me. I haven't gained any weight, but I have maintained the 75 pounds (and still have 1,000 calories a day). It's March 1994, which means that I have kept my weight the same for around four years, the longest I've ever maintained any weight. Up until March 1992, when my uncle sold his business, I worked full-time, forty hours per week. I did this at my low weight, despite many doctors saying that I should not even be strong enough to walk. I am totally,

100 percent, self-sufficient. I do not ask for, nor accept, anything from anyone.

I have been unemployed since I stopped working for my uncle. Although I am capable of performing any office work, and doing it much better than many people, I have been unable to find a new job. I don't look that much. I know I'm capable. People who know me, or those I have worked with, also know I am capable. However, a total stranger is going to look at me and not want to risk hiring me. Although I could be wrong, I'm pretty sure it's because of my appearance. "You look as though you have AIDS," I've been told on a few occasions. This shows how foolish some people can be. They think I have AIDS, only because it's the "disease of the '90s." If these were the 1940s, people would assume that I had just returned from a concentration camp. Well, my attitude is that they're stupid, I don't need them, and it's their loss.

Although I have been unemployed for a long time, I had previously saved enough money to last me for a while. After all, my only "real" expense is my rent. It's not as though I have a huge bill for food (thirty to thirty-five dollars per month), and I don't do anything in the way of entertainment.

In one sense, my life is similar to the way it was in Massachusetts. I pretty much spend my days doing nothing. At my mother's request, I call home at seven-thirty in the morning, every day, seven days per week, fifty-two weeks per year. ("So I know you're alive," she tells me. "I worry so much.") Once every four weeks, I go to the library and check out some books, attempting to concentrate on them. Sometimes I'm successful, sometimes not. Once per week, I go to the supermarket. When my mother visits, I usually get out more. I'll walk around the malls with her or just keep her company. However, there is one difference—I am on my own. My mom comes to visit from December to March (she likes to get away from the snow), but even then, I am still on my own. Also, I have not been vegetating these past few months. I've been writing this book.

Another improvement is that in addition to maintaining the 75 pounds, I am much less preoccupied and obsessed with thoughts of food and weight. Furthermore, I don't care if I live or die. This apathy about life may not be good, but it's better than an intense wish to die.

I'll finish my story with a few random thoughts.

I'm hungry twenty-four hours per day, around the clock, whether I'm awake or asleep, all the time. However, even though I'm constantly hungry, and my stomach is always growling, I'm not sure if I ever actually "want" to eat.

Sometimes, I think this whole anorexia issue started as a game ten years ago and just got out of hand. I received no lack of attention, but maybe I wanted more. Perhaps to begin with, I did this for attention, and one thing led to another. Maybe if so-and-so had or had not done such and such a thing, none of this would have happened. However, it's all in the past now.

Sometimes I think that the anorexia is still a game (a very stupid and foolish one)—or even a contest. I'm 99 percent sure that it's my way of feeling in control of myself. I also know that my greatest fear of ever gaining weight, even just a couple of pounds, is that I would lose all my willpower and self-control, and not be able to stop.

Sometimes, I think if I started feeling skinny, I wouldn't even realize it—maybe won't even allow myself to feel skinny. Perhaps I'm scared to get better or don't even want to. I've been this way for so long, I don't know of any other way to live. It's as though for some reason, I'm holding on to the anorexia and don't want to let go. The anorexia is my shield, protecting me from something.

I don't think doctors know what they're doing, at least in the case of most of the ones I've been to—Nauss, Wiener, and Spielberg excluded. I feel that my experiences with different therapists speak for themselves. Many doctors say that the key to getting better is to gain weight, so that I will have a clear mind to work on the depression. They say my mind cannot function at such a low weight. My question to them is "If this is true, how did I get all A's in school, work forty hours per week, and write this book?" Other doctors say the key is to snap out of the depression, so that I'll have the motivation to get better and the desire to live. I don't know which is the correct answer. Actually, I don't think there is a right one. I believe the bottom line is that everyone is different and needs to be treated as an individual.

I have not had a psychiatrist since moving to Florida, and no longer see a physician for any kind of checkup.

As far as the future is concerned, I don't know what to think. I do not feel skinny or fat, happy or sad, optimistic or pessimistic. I don't care if I live or die. I have no feelings at all. I also have no expectations of getting better, because I make no attempt. But who knows? Maybe one day I'll wake up with a whole new attitude and snap out of the anorexia and depression just like that. Anything's possible.

I take it one day at a time. I still think of fasting, but tell myself, "Have your 1,000 calories today. You can always starve yourself starting tomorrow." Although I have no plans, I believe it's only a matter of time before I do fast to death (maybe in a week, maybe ten years from now, or maybe not at all–I don't know).

No matter what happens, I will get better only when I decide to get better. Michael Krasnow has to make the first step. No one is going to make me better. It's in my hands, completely up to me.

If nothing else comes of this book, at least it has kept me busy and helped to pass the time. Who knows? Maybe it will be a major development. Maybe it will become a best-seller, and as I said in Chapter 1, lead to a greater awareness not only of anorexia, but male anorexia. Maybe other ten- or twelve-year-old boys who feel fat will read this book and find it of some help. Maybe doctors who read this book will have a better understanding of what goes through an anorexic's mind and be able to offer more help to a patient. Maybe. . . Life is full of Maybe's.

Epilogue I

Well, I found a publisher–The Haworth Press. Today is July 25, 1995. Since over a year has gone by since I finished my story, I decided to add an epilogue. After all, unless you borrowed this book from a library or a friend, are reading it in the aisles of a bookstore, or obtained a copy some other way, you just used your money to buy the story of my life, and it's only fair that you be given a complete, up-to-date story.

Everything is basically the same. I'm still 75 pounds, still have 1,000 calories per day, still don't care if I live or die, etc., etc. In other words, I still exist, but nothing else; and as I've said all along, it's only a matter of time until I fast and starve myself to death.

There are two significant differences. Remember Jason, the one who was "more like a brother than a cousin"? Well, he and a few of the people with whom he works started a finance company, and they asked me to run it for them. I guess it's the ideal job. The location and hours couldn't be better. All I need to do is walk across the street from my apartment to get to my office. I work three days per week, about five hours each day. Even without this location and these hours, I still couldn't ask for a better job. You see, the company has just started and is understandably very small. Although I put in only fifteen-or-so hours per week, I'm able to do all the work myself. Therefore, I'm the only employee and can make my own rules. I'm in charge, dress however I feel like dressing, work whenever I feel like working, and do whatever I feel like doing.

Other than my new job, which started in April 1994, there's been only one other change. Not too long ago, I made a spur-of-the-moment decision to become my own guardian. I called my lawyer in Massachusetts, he went through the paperwork, and on July 17 (just last week), I was given back my guardianship.

This brings my story to a close. There's nothing else I can think of telling you. Just let me say that if you think you have anorexia nervosa–or know someone who has it–and would like to get in touch with me for any reason, you're more than welcome to write. My address is 1776 Polk Street, #159, Hollywood, FL 33020. Unless something unforeseen happens (e.g., I become famous and receive thousands of letters), I promise to answer everyone. If you're willing to take the time to write, then it's the least I can do. I'm not going to offer any cures, but sometimes it's nice just being able to communicate with someone who has at least some idea of how you feel. It would be great if I could be of help to anyone, in any way–even just as a listening board.

Epilogue II

Well, here we go again–another epilogue. I really don't feel like doing this, but the people at The Haworth Press wanted me to answer a few questions. They say you'll want to know what I eat (a typical ten-day period is at the end of this epilogue), what I do during the day, etc., etc. So, I agreed to write this.

It's March 1996, and except for the following two changes, everything's the same. First, I'm not working anymore. I didn't stop for any special reason, I just no longer felt like working. I'm not looking for a new job–simply waiting for this book to get published. Second, my mom is now a permanent resident of Florida. She is living in an apartment about ten minutes from me.

As for how I spend my time, there's not a lot to tell you. I do some reading during the day, and turn on the television for an hour or so in the evening. I could have kept a diary for you, but that seemed pointless. I mean, if I had sat on my porch for two hours (I live on the eleventh floor and do a lot of people watching), would I have said that at 1:30 p.m. I stood up to stretch?

Variations in my day would include walking to the market (once a week), going to the library (once a month), doing my laundry (once every two or three weeks), and visits from my mom or Neil (he lives in Miami–about thirty minutes from me). I'm not saying there isn't anything else I do; I'm giving you just the basics. One thing to keep in mind is that my inactivity has nothing to do with my strength or energy. It's because a lot of the time, I just don't feel like doing anything. When I have something that needs to be done, I do it.

Now, I'll finish with a few in-no-order comments. The Haworth Press wanted my book to have a list of eating-disorders organizations, places where people could (supposedly) get help. I refused to allow this. You see, I don't believe in these places, and felt it would have been hypocritical of me to include them in my book.

Another item The Haworth Press and I discussed was having my mother make a short contribution to my book. I was not strongly opposed to this, but I did have misgivings, and decided against it. I guess I felt that each item added to my story by somebody else (I had already compromised by allowing Dr. Spielberg and Dr. Wiener to make some comments) would take away from it being my book.

When I asked my mom what she would have written, her response was that she would mainly just stress that family—especially the parents—should always be supportive and always be there.

This second epilogue was not written very well, but as I said at the beginning, I didn't feel like writing this, and put very little effort into it. The end.

*   *   *

The Haworth Press wanted me to tell you what I eat. I said that I couldn't really do this because there are no set rules. I make it a point to vary what I have, and won't commit to anything. Also, I used to be obsessed with thinking about food and about what I was going to eat. Now that I'm no longer preoccupied with these thoughts, I don't like to make a big deal about what I have.

Eventually, although I had my doubts, I agreed to write up a sample ten-day period. Now that I'm including this, I'll probably get lots of advice from "expert" nutritionists about what I should or should not be doing, what I should or should not change, etc., etc.

In the morning, I take one multivitamin, an iron supplement, and five amino-acid tablets. In the evening, I take another iron supplement and five more amino-acid tablets. I have no idea whether or not these do anything for me.

The following is just a sample. It doesn't mean this is what I have all the time, or that I never have anything else. Again, it's just a sample.

	Morning	Evening
Day one	2 oz. cereal (Total, Frosted Flakes, whatever) milk	peanut butter sandwich banana juice
Day two	2 oz. cereal milk	peanut butter sandwich banana juice
Day three	2 oz. cereal milk	peanut butter sandwich banana juice
Day four	2 oz. cereal milk	Heinz vegetarian beans juice
Day five	2 oz. cereal milk	Heinz vegetarian beans juice
Day six	2 oz. cereal milk	tuna fish sandwich with mayonnaise juice
Day seven	2 oz. cereal milk	tuna fish sandwich with mayonnaise juice
Day eight	1 1/2 granola bars chocolate milk	peanut butter sandwich can of corn juice
Day nine	1 1/2 granola bars chocolate milk	peanut butter sandwich can of pineapple juice
Day ten	1 1/2 granola bars chocolate milk	peanut butter sandwich can of pineapple juice

Editor's note: The amount of each item consumed varies from day to day, but stays within the limit of 1,000 calories.

Appendix I

A Psychiatrist's Comments

As a physician and a psychiatrist, I don't think that there is anything that is more difficult to prepare oneself for than the self-starvation that occurs in anorexic patients. There is some possibility that one is slightly more prepared to tolerate the dieting frenzy that may occur in adolescent females more so than when this occurs in males. Michael was not my patient when he first started to have difficulties with his eating disorder, but his symptoms clearly presented in a classical way with severe restriction of intake, progressive development of symptoms of feeling that he was fat, difficulty in terms of accepting his need for treatment, and associated depressive and obsessive-compulsive symptoms. The presence of his toothbrushing and his preoccupation with studying were symptoms of his obsessive-compulsive-type problems; and his several suicide attempts, although they were by starvation, probably did occur in conjunction with co-existing major depressive symptoms.

When I first met Michael, I had already heard of him from the nursing staff in regard to his weight and his general appearance and their overall concerns about his health. It is remarkable that Michael's physical health has persisted in spite of his severe malnutrition and persistent self-starvation. Throughout the time that I was actively treating Michael, my primary concerns focused on his insistence on maintaining his weight at such a low level that prevented any opportunity for him to have enough leeway in his diet to be adequately nourished at any point in time.

At various times I had attempted to get him to increase his overall caloric intake, even if it meant that he would then exercise some to try to limit his weight gain. I had told him at that time that I felt that it would be more possible for him to have some type of adequate nutrition if he were eating 1,000 calories per day, and burning 250 calories through exercise, than [eating] what appeared to be a very meager 750 calories per day.[1] In general, adequate dietary intake for him is based on a 2,000+ calorie-per-day diet for someone weighing in the neighborhood of 130 pounds; Michael was eating slightly more than one-third of that.

During each of his admissions, there were always numerous lab values that were markedly abnormal, but Michael continued to refuse to increase his caloric intake even to normalize some of his lab values and reduce the risk of the chronic health-related problems that I was so concerned about. His refusal persisted even when he started to have some degeneration of his liver in a type of self-cannibalistic attempt by his body to maintain itself during his severe starvation episodes.

I had first learned of Michael's intent to write this book approximately two years ago when I spoke to the patient's mother. I had called her place of employment without knowing that she was working there. Michael's mother had informed me that Michael was starting to write a book and had been looking for a publishing company willing to work with him. Approximately nine months later, I received an initial draft of Michael's attempt to describe his experience as an anorexic.

It is very clear that one of Michael's unique characteristics is his perseverance. He used this initial effort to further describe both the general experiences of being an anorexic as well as to describe his own individual experiences. The second draft I received from him subsequently included the request to add some psychiatric perspective on Michael's experience. His second draft was much better written, organized, and meaningful to me as it presented the experiences that Michael had been through with me as his psychiatrist. His earlier effort seemed more like an extended diary. Michael clearly has recognized the

---

1. Author's note: I do not recall having ever been on a 750-calorie-per-day diet.

extent to which he needed to expand his account of his experiences in order to allow his readers to recognize the pain and suffering that he had experienced and that most anorexics encounter in the course of their struggles with this eating disorder.

I was especially impressed with the extensive material Michael had included in this draft—personal accounts of his difficulties when his father was dying as well as after his father's death. Michael has shared with readers details that had not even been disclosed in therapy with me. Michael is certainly a unique person, even in terms of being a male anorexic, which is fairly uncommon. It is apparent that there may be more male bulimics in adolescence than male anorexics. Even as an anorexic, Michael is unusual since he has limited his weight solely by food restriction. Frequently, anorexics involve other methods to control their weight, including taking laxatives or emetics to induce vomiting or using diuretics or enemas to help lose weight or reduce weight gain.

It would perhaps be helpful if I included some of the diagnostic criteria for anorexia nervosa. These criteria are taken from the latest *Diagnostic and Statistical Manual in Psychiatry*, known as DSM-IV. The onset usually occurs between the ages of 10 and 30—after the age of menarche in women and possibly after puberty in males. The rate of onset increases rapidly in the teenage years, with the maximum frequency occurring from 17 to 20 years of age. About 85 percent of all anorexics have their onset of illness between 13 and 20, and frequently these patients have had a history of eating difficulties in the past.

Patients often refuse to eat in public or in front of others—even including their families—and try to lose weight by decreasing any high-calorie carbohydrate or fatty foods.

Perhaps it would be helpful to have a table that includes the specific diagnostic criteria that apply for anorexia nervosa. These are primarily directed toward women, although under Item D where absence of menstrual cycle often occurs in women, there is also often a decrease in testosterone and sexual drive in males.

DIAGNOSTIC CRITERIA FOR ANOREXIA NERVOSA

Item A. Refusal to maintain body weight at or above normal weight expected, or failure to gain weight during a period of growth, leading to a body weight less than 85 percent of normal.

Item B. Intense fear of gaining weight or becoming fat even if the person is currently underweight.

Item C. Disturbance in the way in which one's body weight or shape is experienced; undue influence of body weight or shape on self-evaluation; minimization or denial of the seriousness of current low body weight.

Item D. In most postmenarchal females, amenorrhea, i.e., the absence of at least three consecutive menstrual cycles.

There are two specific types of anorexia: one is a restricting type in which the person does not engage in purging behavior, including self-induced vomiting, misuse of laxatives, diuretics, enemas, or use of emetics. There is also a binge-eating and purging type: the person regularly engages in excessive amounts of bingeing with subsequent purging, which may be self-induced vomiting or use of emetics or misuse of laxatives, diuretics, or enemas.

In both types of disorder, although more frequently in anorexia nervosa, there is often an excessive use of exercise as a way to limit weight gain or to actually reduce weight.

Patients frequently are first diagnosed due to physical symptoms that may accompany their anorexia, since they do not view their weight loss as a symptom or illness. Frequently, they may develop hypothermia (low body temperature), edema due to low protein in their bloodstream, bradycardia (slow heart rate), low blood pressure, and various other metabolic problems due to poor nutrition. These include anemia, changes in the pH of their blood, and inability to excrete fluid through their kidneys. They may have changes in their EKGs and various other problems due to their dietary restriction; also these may be complicated by treatment due to their intolerance of rapid increases in dietary intake, fluid protein, or salt.

Other medical complications frequently include general wasting and reduced thyroid metabolism, cold intolerance, and difficulty maintaining body temperature. Cardiac problems may include arrhythmias, atrial and ventricular premature contractions, slow heart rate, rapid heart rate (known as ventricular tachycardia), and possible death due to ventricular tachycardia. There are digestive problems, including gastric dilatation, bloating, constipation, and pain. There are reproductive problems with low levels of reproductive hormones, loss of menstrual cycle, and reduced sex drive. There are hematologic problems, including bone marrow-related depression with reduced output of white cells and red cells, subsequently increasing the risk of infection and anemia. There are psychiatric problems, including depression and difficulty thinking; and there also can be health risks caused by hypoglycemia. There are risks of seizures from other changes in fluid balance and general fatigue and weakness.

In regard to Michael, he certainly experienced multiple examples of these problems, including hypothermia and cardiac difficulties due to slow heart rate; he did experience two episodes of respiratory arrest in which he stopped breathing. Michael also experienced probable seizure-like activity as a result of his severe hypoglycemia on two occasions, and even had hypoglycemia while he had been on an IV fluid regimen, which had preceded his respiratory arrests. He had bone marrow problems that required relatively extensive treatment with high-potency steroids to cause his bone marrow to produce red cells and white cells.

In regard to describing my work with Michael, there are two phases of Michael's treatment, and these overlapped to some extent. The first phase occurred during his initial hospitalizations and probably extended through the time that his father died from Lou Gehrig's disease. Michael was very resistant to treatment or medication most of that time, although more resistant to treatment than he was to medication. By treatment, I probably mean that he would not agree to gain or maintain weight. He had initially gained some weight, and as he points out in regard to his experience at Children's Hospital, he probably could have maintained his weight at some point in the low 90s. It was a very complicated process to try to negotiate with Michael about what he was willing or not willing to do. I had my own difficulties in trying to refer Michael to *any* eating disorder specialist due to each specialist's own preconceived minimum weight that he had to achieve before they would even agree to evaluate, much less treat, him. Each specialist required that Michael gain weight up to 100, 110, or 115 pounds as part of some rigid orientation of a safety margin for Michael in regard to his physical well-being before any specialized eating disorder treatment units would agree to see him. This included both inpatient and outpatient specialists. This seemed unfair to Michael in terms of denying him specialty care by eating disorder specialists because he was unwilling to gain the required minimum weight to be permitted to get treatment from specialists. It was then up to me (and I am not an eating disorder specialist) to try to deal with Michael in terms of his eating disorder problems without the benefit of the expertise of people with specific training in eating disorders. This also was unfair to Michael in relation to the extent to which he had been able to maintain his weight at a very low level for an extended period of time without major health-related consequences. It appeared that the eating disorder specialists wanted some reassurance that Michael was going to participate actively in treatment by making a concession in regard to his initial starting weight for any further treatment to occur. They also demanded that he agree to gain additional weight even beyond the weight that he was expected to gain initially in order to be accepted for treatment. This situation left Dr. Spielberg and me scratching our heads and very frustrated with the renowned eating disorder programs in the Boston area, which consistently refused to treat the patient due to his unwillingness to initially commit to both gaining weight in order to be accepted for treatment and to continue to gain weight in treatment. It seemed a kind of self-selection by the experts[2] to treat only those patients

---

2. Author's note: Although I would not call these doctors "experts," I think Dr. Wiener should be congratulated for his criticism of them.

who were already willing to accept treatment, rather than direct-ing their expertise toward increasing the level of cooperation with patients who have not already made that commitment to allow themselves to gain weight.

Michael has certainly amazed anyone who has treated him, probably by his ability to tolerate his incredibly low body weight for as long as he has. I am very surprised that he has not experi-enced more complications in relation to cardiac, respiratory, kidney, or liver-related problems than he already has. It appears that he has maintained a very fragile equilibrium in his body so that it has not persisted in self-cannibalizing itself in order to maintain his existence. There have been numerous episodes of complications associated with his weight dropping even below 75 pounds. I was clearly certain that Michael would not survive when his weight had dropped to 67 pounds, which was approxi-mately one-half his ideal body weight of 135 pounds. Michael clearly was one of the most challenging patients I have ever treated because of the severity of his eating disorder, the difficul-ties that he had in accepting treatment, and not allowing himself to be dependent on anyone other than himself. In addition, his general obsessive style of thinking probably compounded his difficulties in terms of giving up his rituals about eating. Clearly, most of the things that Michael describes about his being able to surreptitiously disguise his food restriction were known to me, and I believe that this was something that he was challenged by when he was put in the hospital against his will. He obviously had more ability to overcome any obstacles that we placed in his way as far as his efforts at food restriction and weight loss. Michael did always seem to have an interest in wanting to get better, but it always had to be on his terms, and attempting to restrict his activities or behavior in order to try to increase his compliance was always met with a lack of success and even greater resistance and noncooperation. Any coercive attempts almost always, in retrospect, produced some type of backlash on Michael's part to cancel out any gains.

The best example of this kind of physical backlash on Michael's part was when he had been briefly tube-fed. In spite of his head being restrained, Michael was still somehow able to shake his head from side to side violently enough to throw the feeding tube back up his throat from his stomach. I don't think that I have ever seen any psychiatric patient resist treatment in a more intense or self-destructive way than this experience when Michael weighed 67 pounds. It is interesting that Michael subsequently became more cooperative, I believe, when he recognized how great a loss it would be for his mother if he died so soon after his father's death. Michael continued to have difficulty accepting treatment whenever it was offered, but it had never been so great as during that hospitalization when he had a respiratory arrest, several hypoglycemic seizures, and bone marrow depression requiring steroid treatment.

Recently I have had some additional contact with Michael's mother. I believe Michael and his mother have established some improved relationship with each other, although their relationship was never bad. Michael seems to have progressed from working for his uncle in Florida to trying to express himself through his current book. He is certainly making an effort to share his experiences as an anorexic patient with other patients who are anorexic and, as he hopes himself, with therapists who treat anorexic patients.

It was clearly an honor to be asked by Michael for my impressions of the story of his life with anorexia. I had communicated earlier to Michael's mother my feeling that Michael's initial draft was more preliminary and needed more of Michael's personal experiences and personal perspective on those experiences. This book reflects the Michael that I knew and worked with over those years. I worked with Michael approximately three and half years, and during that time he taught me a great deal about his sense of perseverance and determination. I always tried to work with Michael in relation to his own needs. Michael is one of a group of patients who I have worked with over a period of time, primarily in inpatient settings, who have a history of a poor response to past treatment. The majority of other patients are probably those who have been through childhood trauma and abuse, and have been very mistrustful of treatment in general and men in particular. There is no evidence that Michael himself had any psychological or physical trauma during his childhood, but he is representative of a group of patients who have difficulty accepting treatment. Through treating patients with post-traumatic stress disorder, the psychological illness that frequently occurs after abuse, I have learned a great deal about how to work with patients in regard to making them feel part of the treatment. By the time Michael left Massachusetts and moved to Florida, this process had improved to some extent, but had not stabilized. This is indicated by his food restriction whenever his mother was not living at home with him.

Apparently, Michael subsequently was able to balance his self-starvation and his need for help while in Florida. He continued to work for his uncle over a period of time and apparently has not experienced any of the dire complications that one would predict by his being only at 55 percent of his ideal body weight. The real lesson I have learned from working with Michael and with other patients suffering from eating disorders, other more common psychiatric conditions, or post-traumatic stress disorder, is that the therapist needs to be very accepting with patients like Michael in order to gain their trust and improve their ability to live productive lives. I believe that Michael did accomplish this by moving to Florida and by working for his uncle, and that he has taken another significant step forward by writing this book and by then working diligently to find a publisher. I am glad that he has the opportunity to write this book and to see it published. Hopefully this will give him some new opportunity to express himself and possibly to improve his physical condition as well as to cope better with his problem with self-starvation and all of its meanings to him.

The other significant element that I have learned from working with Michael and his mother concerns the difficulties that a parent has in seeing a child with such an insidious psychiatric disorder. Michael's mother, Gail, is also a very special person, and all of Michael's praise within the book is probably well deserved. It was very heartening to me as a psychiatrist to see how caring she was toward Michael, even in the face of her husband's approaching death and subsequent to his death. I believe that there is a perseverance in his mother as well, that was a big part of sustaining Michael, even when he didn't want to live. I would suggest that Michael's calls to his family when he ran away several times were in fact an acknowledgment on his part of how much her caring meant to him.

Clearly, this story indicates how important it is to people such as Michael not to lose the support and caring of their family or their professional treaters while experiencing psychiatric problems. I am hopeful that the kind of dialogue that Michael was able to develop and sustain with his mother during his multiple crises and admissions related to his eating disorder may be encouragement to family members of patients with eating disorders or other psychiatric disorders to reestablish some type of renewed involvement to the benefit of both the patient and the family. When families reject individuals such as Michael, it is not helpful either to the family or to the person himself or herself. Michael is certainly someone who has been sustained by his relationship with his mother more than anything else.

I treated Michael with multiple selective serotonin reuptake inhibitors (such as Prozac, Zoloft, and Paxil) for his eating disorder, but none of these were effective. Similarly, they were not very effective in regard to his depression. Such drugs are often significantly effective for a large percentage of such patients. It emphasizes the ultimate value of caring by the people taking care of Michael and by his family that seemed to sustain him through the worst parts of his eating disorder. His relationship with his father had apparently been very important to him when he was younger, but due to the father's illness, Michael became somewhat more distant from him during the father's last illness.[3] This was partly because Michael undoubtedly felt that he had been a strain to his father and even blamed himself for the rapidity with

---

3. Author's note: Even though I agree with most (not all) of Dr. Wiener's comments, this is not true. I did not become more distant from my father, and I don't know why Dr. Wiener says that I did. Of course, this is probably one of those instances of the doctor knowing how the patient feels better than the patient does.

which he died from Lou Gehrig's disease. Perhaps Michael anticipated his father's rapid downhill course and death more clearly than anyone else. Michael's relationship with his brother, although somewhat intermittent, also remained very strong and sustaining, and I believe that Neil did a great deal to reinforce Michael's sense of connection to his family when Michael and his mother were having difficulty maintaining that sense of connection themselves.

In regard to general treatment for eating disorders, I am a strong advocate of patients with significant eating disorders being assessed for co-existing psychiatric disturbances, including obsessive-compulsive disorder and depression. The possibility of sometimes treating these other related conditions with antidepressants may reduce the patient's difficulty in terms of engaging in treatment. The possibility also exists, specifically for the serotonin reuptake inhibitors, to be directly helpful for the eating disorder itself. The most commonly known antidepressant for eating disorder is Prozac, although in my experience Paxil has also been very helpful to patients with eating disorder symptoms, especially if they also manifest symptoms of depression or obsessive-compulsive disorder. Other serotonin reuptake inhibitors that have been frequently used in depression are Zoloft and Effexor, but it is less clear that these drugs have specific benefits in the treatment of eating disorders. The general evidence supports that a great deal needs to be done in terms of research and additional clarification of types of eating disorders and patterns of response to medication and treatment. Michael's book adds a personal element, revealing the difficulties such patients have in accepting treatment and the pain these conditions impose on the patients and their families. Hopefully, Michael's book on his experience as an eating disorder patient will increase people's awareness of the problem that anorexia nervosa represents to its sufferers and their families.

Stephen R. Wiener, MD

Appendix II

Discharge Summaries

BOURNEWOOD HOSPITAL
Name of Institution

Name KRASNOW, Michael   **No.** 42708

Date. ADM: 03/15/88
DIS: 04/13/88

DISCHARGE SUMMARY

The patient is an 18-year-old, white, Jewish, single male who was admitted to Bournewood Hospital for extreme malnutrition, anorexia nervosa, and an attempt to starve himself to death. The patient apparently has had a four-year history of anorexia nervosa originally manifested by some obsessional rituals. He had been treated at Westwood Lodge by Dr. B. He had continued to be in treatment with Dr. P until January or February of 1987. The patient states that there was really no improvement in his condition during his time of treatment with Dr. P. The patient then had essentially been out of treatment for a period of time until he was hospitalized at Emerson Hospital in October of 1987. His weight had been dropping, and he was apparently making some kind of plan to run away to starve himself to death. He had apparently then eloped from Emerson Hospital to Florida and had made a number of phone calls back to his mother in Boston, and she had somehow succeeded in tracing him to Florida where he was placed in custody by police and transferred back to Boston. He was hospitalized at St. Elizabeth's Hospital for an additional period of time, essentially left the hospital in a relatively unstable state, and had really not been in treatment subsequently and had been gradually losing weight. His weight had drifted down to approximately 82 pounds prior to admission, and it is difficult to determine the exact motivation that he has for maintaining his weight at this low level. He had apparently again been making plans to run away and starve himself to death, and had both bus information and hotel information for Dallas, Texas. At his state of malnutrition it would only have taken three to four days probably for him to die by self-starvation, and it was fortunate that he was hospitalized at this time.

Following his admission here, he was initially very resistant but passively compliant in a number of different ways. He did ultimately agree to take amoxapine 200 mg per day, which seemed to decrease the intensity of some of his wish to starve himself. There was no overall additional antidepressant effect and no other side effect of the medication that was notable. The patient's weight fluctuated between 80 and 81 pounds, and the patient was quite adamant about his unwillingness to gain weight. He did, however, agree to consideration of finding an outpatient therapist, but was convinced that they would allow him to remain at his current weight rather than insist on his gaining weight. His immediate need to starve himself to death seemed to dissipate somewhat also, but he was not motivated for actual treatment of his eating disorder. There was some consideration about whether this represented some connection to his grandfather who had died four years ago and to what extent the grandfather had been cachectic before his death. The patient denied any connection to his grandfather, and it may be that the actuality of his eating disorder and the condition of the grandfather himself prior to his death may have been entirely coincidental. The patient himself seemed to have a very severe eating disorder, with all of the usual preoccupations about looking fat, controlled dietary intake, and the insistence of the normality of his low weight. The patient did manifest some depressive symptomatology, but was otherwise more in the category of an eating disorder or an obsessive-compulsive personality than a major depression. The antidepressant was primarily for his obsessive preoccupation with his weight and other obsessions that he had.

PAST PSYCHIATRIC TREATMENT: As stated, he has been in three other psychiatric hospitals: Westwood Lodge in 1983, Emerson and St. Elizabeth's in 1987.

PAST MEDICAL HISTORY: The patient apparently had been relatively healthy up until he began to become more and more obsessed in 1983 with toothbrushing rituals and other cognitive obsessions.

FAMILY HISTORY: The patient states that there are some difficulties within the family due to a relatively poor relationship with his brother and the patient states that he often feels very jealous and competitive with other people, and [he] also feels that this is related to his eating disorder. He feels that if he were on an eating disorders unit he would be competitive with other anorexics about maintaining his weight at a low level. He was unable to comment about whether if they were gaining weight that he would try to outgain their weight. He feels that he would be relatively unable to cooperate in a voluntary program.

HOSPITAL COURSE: The patient gradually adjusted to the unit, did agree to antidepressants, and was cooperative in individual therapy. He, however, remained very resistant to [his] need to gain weight, his willingness to participate in an eating disorder program, and his ability to contract about his maintaining the weight that he gained while in the hospital.

LABORATORY TESTS AND VITAL SIGNS: [Tests] indicated an initial period of dehydration which gradually compensated. General hyperthermia, which was more common in the afternoon, was treated mainly with bedrest. The patient was on some type of food monitoring while he was here but was generally uncooperative to any food supplements or any kind of other supplementation. Ultimately, through coordination by his outside pediatrician, Dr. Alan Nauss, the patient was able to be transferred to the Judge Baker Psychiatric Unit at Children's Hospital for further treatment of his eating disorder. His periods of dehydration, were essentially normal with the exception of an elevated calcium on admission and an elevated parathyroid hormone. He did receive an MRI scan at Faulkner Hospital on 04/11/88, which was reportedly initially normal, but the final report has not been received. This hypercalcemia and parathyroid hormone should continue to be monitored due to the likelihood that this represents an incipient stage of hyperparathyroidism.

FINAL DIAGNOSIS: Anorexia nervosa.
                            Obsessive-compulsive personality disorder.
                            Hyperparathyroidism.

Stephen R. Wiener, MD
D: 04/16/88
T: 04/21/88

The patient is a 19-year-old white, single, Jewish male who had been admitted to Bournewood Hospital on 02/15/88 and discharged on 04/13/88 to Children's Hospital for severe eating disorder. He had subsequently been treated at Children's Hospital from 04/13/88 through 05/24/88, when he escaped and attempted to starve himself in a motel room in Durham, North Carolina. The patient had been 81 pounds when he arrived at Bournewood, did not gain any weight there, but did gain 9 pounds at Children's Hospital prior to his running away from there. During his self-starvation from 05/24/88 to 06/1/88, he lost weight down to 74 pounds, including a moderate amount of dehydration. Subsequent to his return to Massachusetts, by calling his mother and having her pick him up in North Carolina, the patient returned to Newton-Wellesley Hospital. The patient has been in treatment here since that time, but again has not gained any weight. He has practiced a number of tricks to try to convince staff that he was eating when he was not, but this essentially has done nothing but to defeat any efforts to help him gain weight. It appears that his current maintenance calorie requirements due to his state of malnutrition are only in the 700-calorie per day range. The patient keeps stating that he will gain weight, but has been unable to do so.

During the time that he has been in the hospital, proceedings have gone forward to obtain a guardianship with his mother as the guardian of record. The powers sought include those to authorize tube feedings, IV fluids, ECT, and medication. Hopefully, there will be some resolution of this in the very near future, and the patient will start on ECT treatments at Bournewood due to his lack of response to any behavioral program attempted to this point. The patient has been on fluoxetine during the time that he was at Newton-Wellesley Hospital at 40 mg. per day, with some questionable improvement in terms of his overall resistance, but no improvement in terms of his compliance with the treatment program here. The patient agrees that he feels somewhat better and focuses on the issues of his inability and unwillingness to consistently eat. I have discussed with him that there is a major difference between his inability to eat and his unwillingness to eat. We have discussed the necessary factors for him to be more able and more willing consistently in terms of his need for improvement. Particularly, this has been discussed in relation to the possible benefits derived from ECT, and arrangements have been with Dr. N at Bournewood Hospital to attempt to institute such treatment, especially where this may be life-saving in relation to his overall chronic malnutrition.

Interestingly, there have not been any severe, acute medical complications of his severe malnutrition up to this point, although that is somewhat surprising in view of the overall level of his malnutrition. It is possible that to some extent this has been mildly alleviated by his having a history of an elevated calcium, which may have caused some demineralization of his bone. This might reduce his relative weight in relation to his ideal body weight. The patient had had a history of elevated calciums at Bournewood, but this had levelled off apparently when he was at Children's, and he had had a negative ultrasound at Bournewood and a negative MRI scan at Children's Hospital. While at Newton-Wellesley, he had one calcium which was near the upper limits of normal at 10.4 and a normal calcium at 9.5. His parathyroid hormone that was done here, I believe, is still pending at the time of his discharge. He will continue to be followed for the possibility that this represents early parathyroid disease at Bournewood and subsequently.

The patient has been cooperative in terms of trying to arrange his transfer to Bournewood and has seemed willing to allow himself to have ECT as a possible resolution to his short-term inability to gain weight. I have discussed with him his need to maintain and continue to gain weight, but the patient is still very unclear about what his attitudes will be subsequent to his treatments with ECT. He is concerned about the guardianship and the powers granted to his mother, especially in relation to the extent to which that may and will abridge some of his own personal rights in terms of hospitalization, medication, and choice of therapists. I have discussed with him how to this point his mother has really not been an interference with his treatment and has in essence helped him make decisions that were otherwise impossible for him to make due to his ambivalence about himself, his periods of self-starvation, and his preoccupation with not eating. The patient was somewhat relieved about the extent to which the guardianship has gone slowly, and has been more cooperative in terms of revealing some of the difficulties that he has had eating, his subterfuges to try to convince people that he was eating more than he was, and his overall concerns about how he will be viewed by his family if he has the ECT treatments.

His laboratory values, in spite of all his malnutrition, have remained more normal than they have in the past, and it is somewhat reassuring to me in terms of his ability to tolerate the ECT treatments. Opinions have been obtained from Dr. H at Children's Hospital and Dr. A at McLean Hospital in relation to the treatment of patients such as Michael with ECT. Both of them are highly encouraging about the possible outcome, especially the extent to which his condition may actually be some type of atypical or delusional depression, as suggested by Dr. L.

The patient will be transferred to Bournewood Hospital for continued care by Dr. N, and with coordination of his care by myself. We will obtain his guardianship during the week of 06/27/88 if granted by the court, and hopefully, this will present Michael with a different set of circumstances wherein he may be more cooperative due to the fact that feeling that his treatment choices are being made by someone other than himself, so that he really does not have to cooperate by giving his consent in order to gain benefits of such treatments. Overall, his prognosis has to be very guarded to his history of self-starvation and attempted suicide by this means. His condition on discharge would have to be considered unimproved.

FINAL DIAGNOSIS: Anorexia nervosa.
Major depression with psychotic features.
Obsessive-compulsive personality disorder.

Stephen Wiener, MD
D and T: 06/27/88

ADDENDUM

Guardianship was obtained in relation to the transfer to Bournewood Hospital, and patient was agreeable to this transfer. He remained anxious throughout the weekend and was fearful about losing control of his decisions about his care and was very focused on this as an issue, as in any of his other obsessive concerns. He was also concerned about his relationship with me changing as a result of his being under the care of another doctor at Bournewood, and while I explained to him that this would be the case, I also explained to him that as a result of the ECT, he was not going to remember a large amount of the events which occurred there, and that it was unlikely that this would significantly affect our ability to work together in the future. His condition did not change throughout the weekend and would still have to have been considered unimproved at the time of his discharge.

FINAL DIAGNOSIS: Remain the same.

S. Wiener, MD
07/20/88; 07/26/88

	BOURNEWOOD HOSPITAL	
	Name of Institution	

		Date. ADM: 06/30/88
Name KRASNOW, Michael	**No.** 43037	DIS: 07/29/88

DISCHARGE SUMMARY

Michael Krasnow, a 19-year-old, single, white, Jewish male was admitted to Bournewood Hospital for the second time on June 30, 1988 on a section 12 T.C. paper. Mr. Krasnow had been a patient in Newton-Wellesley Psychiatric Unit from June 1st through June 30th. While there, Mr. Krasnow failed to respond to drug-augmented psychotherapy, more recently having been on Prozac. He has a long history of anorexia nervosa, and he had developed a major depression. Mr. Krasnow has had multiple hospitalizations dating back to age 14. He was readmitted to Bournewood on a Substitutive Judgment Treatment Plan, which included guardianship by his mother, Mrs. Gail Krasnow, and included a series of ECT under anesthesia for his depression. The order was given on June 29th by Judge G of the Norfolk Probate Court based on testimony of Dr. Stephen Wiener. Mr. Krasnow's weight had fluctuated around 80 to 81 pounds for several months.

Prior to hospitalization at Newton-Wellesley, he was at Children's Hospital Medical Center and eloped from there. He went to North Carolina, called his family, and was returned to Boston where he was admitted to the Newton-Wellesley Hospital. Mr. Krasnow allegedly eloped in a suicidal attempt, planning not to eat or drink, thus starving himself and ending his life. Mr. Krasnow gained some weight (from 81 to 90 pounds) at Children's Hospital Medical Center. He had previously run away to Florida and had also planned to run away to Dallas prior to his last Bournewood admission. Mr. Krasnow had been at Emerson Hospital in October and November of 1987 and later was at St. Elizabeth's Hospital. He has had a very severe, compulsive per-

113

sonality with depressive symptoms and borderline features. Generally, Mr. Krasnow was unable to cooperate with treatment because of his personality difficulties. During his hospitalization at Bournewood, he was on Asendin 200 mg at bedtime with no complications and no lifting of his depression, although his cooperation increased relative to eating.

PAST HISTORY: Mr. Krasnow had no clear onset of his illness except that it appeared to coincide with his grandfather's death following cancer. It was unclear to what extent this grandfather, with whom the patient had been very close, had cachexia as a complication of his cancer. The onset also coincided with general adolescent problems, and Mr. Krasnow had difficulty through school feeling that he did not fit in. In spite of this he did very well there and started Babson College, and had been doing very well, especially in Math, prior to his admission to Emerson Hospital last year. He was at Westwood Lodge at age 14 with the onset of severe obsessive-compulsive rituals following his grandfather's death. Subsequently, Mr. Krasnow was an outpatient under the care of Dr. P in Framingham. He stopped that treatment in February, 1987. Subsequently, Mr. Krasnow's weight dwindled and his functioning became impaired. He weighed about 90 pounds when he went to Emerson Hospital.

FAMILY HISTORY: Mr. Krasnow has significant family history. His father was overweight and his mother was moderately overweight. Mr. Krasnow's father had lost a considerable amount of weight since the development several years ago of amyotrophic lateral sclerosis. This illness has been rapidly progressive and Mr. Krasnow has been wheelchair-bound. The patient's mother, Gail, was cooperative with the treatment plan, but it is apparent that she has lived in a highly stressed family. Allegedly, there was some history of some type of childhood seizures on the part of the older brother, and it is unclear what the etiology of these seizures was. There was also question of whether the patient feels to blame for the seizures. It is unclear whether the patient feels guilty about the multiple family illnesses. There was no clear-cut precipitant other than the patient's difficulty in starting college in the fall of 1987.

MEDICAL HISTORY: Mr. Krasnow has had an elevated calcium while at Bournewood, and this was elevated by repeat examination. He also had an elevated parathyroid hormone, an elevated ionized calcium. An ultrasound while at Bournewood and an MRI at Children's Hospital Medical Center were both negative, and it was unclear what the status of his hyperparathyroidism was.

MENTAL STATUS: Mental status on admission revealed a tall, extremely pale, markedly cachectic adult male. He was extremely slow in speech. His affect and underlying mood were markedly depressed. He had fair eye contact throughout the interview but part of the time his eyes were downcast. He was oriented for time, place, and person. There was no gross evidence of any delusions or hallucinations. His judgment was poor. He was in contact with reality. He had some minimal insight into his situation. His general fund of knowledge was within normal limits.

The initial diagnostic impression was major depression with anorexia nervosa, obsessive-compulsive personality disorder.

HOSPITAL COURSE: Mr. Krasnow was admitted to the Male Intensive Care Unit. ECT had previously been discussed with him and it was re-discussed. He had been cleared medically for ECT by his internist at Newton-Wellesley, Dr. Spielberg. He was placed on a regular diet to be weighed daily. In addition, chocolate Ensure was ordered on a prn basis. No neuroleptics or antidepressants were planned. ECT was re-explained to Mr. Krasnow and also to his guardian, who signed the permit for ECT. Mr. Krasnow received his first ECT bilateral with Brevital and Anectine anesthesia on July 1, 1988. That treatment and all subsequent treatments were uneventful. In all, Mr. Krasnow received a total of 13 ECTs, the last of which was given on 07/29/88. The patient's response to ECT was slow and steady, with gradual lifting of his depression, but no improvement in his eating habits. His father was hospitalized on July 6, 1988 as a result of his amyotrophic lateral sclerosis. His condition was terminal, and he expired on July 7, 1988. Mr. Krasnow was given permission to leave the hospital to be with his father at the time of his death, and he participated in the funeral services on July 10th, and two days of memorial week. He became appropriately depressed following his father's death. This depression was soon alleviated with further ECT. Mr. Krasnow was generally resistant to the Adult Program, repeatedly declining to attend adult group therapy. He did participate, however, in the AT Program. Toward the end of his hospitalization Mr. Krasnow met with Dr. Wiener, his mother, and the social worker. It was agreed that Dr. Wiener would follow Mr. Krasnow after hospitalization for supportive psychotherapy. Mr. Krasnow was discharged to the care of his mother on 07/29/88 to return home. His weight at that time was approximately 85 to 87 pounds. His depression had abated and he was considering the possibility of looking for work, possibly returning to a job in the library. He expressed no desire to return to school.

DISCHARGE DIAGNOSIS: (1) Major depression.
                       (2) Anorexia nervosa.
                       (3) Obsessive-compulsive personality.

CONDITION ON DISCHARGE: Mr. Krasnow's condition on discharge was improved to the extent that he was no longer depressed. He had not, however, significantly altered his eating habits, his marked concern about gaining weight, and his feeling that he would be "very fat" over 90 pounds. He will require close monitoring to check on his depression and his overall physical condition. This will be done by Dr. Wiener. If possible, he should return to work.

Dr. N
D: 08/12/88
T: 08/13/88

The patient is a 20-year-old, very emaciated, white male who was readmitted to Newton-Wellesley Hospital for severe weight loss, persistent depression, obsessive-compulsive disorder, and oppositional behavior in relation to eating.

The patient had been treated at Newton-Wellesley, Children's, and Bournewood hospitals last year for a severe episode of weight loss when the patient had lost down to approximately 70 pounds at one point when he had run away to North Carolina and attempted to starve himself in a motel. He had returned to Newton-Wellesley Hospital, had been medically stabilized, and had been subsequently treated with electroconvulsive therapy with a period of seven months of improvement subsequent to his father's death in July 1988 due to rapidly progressive amyotrophic lateral sclerosis. The patient had apparently been losing weight over a period of time from approximately 88 pounds down to 74 pounds at present. He had apparently become increasingly resolute about starving himself to death. It appears that his difficulties had become more significant since Father's Day, his family moving to a new house, and increasing difficulty in relationship with his mother. She is trying to help him cope with the loss of his father and his generalized identity problems and his eating disorder. The mother had also returned to work somewhat recently, and it may have been this actual separation between the patient and his mother by both of them working more full-time that has intensified his problems about eating. The patient himself had started a full-time job approximately at the same time that his weight loss became more substantial, and I feel that this may be related.

The patient had also been switched from Prozac to Anafranil with some anticipation of improvement in approximately November or December, but he apparently did not do better and had some difficulties with urinary retention and a falling white count, decreased platelets, and decreased hematocrit. Initially the feeling was that this may have been related to the Anafranil, but his continued weight loss tended to suggest it was more a result of malnutrition than any other immediate cause. The patient also had some increased liver function tests prior to his admission to Newton-Wellesley Hospital, initially attributed to the Anafranil as well, but I believe they were related to some autolysis of his liver related to the severity of his malnutrition.

The patient is to be admitted for further treatment of his self-starvation, his anorexia nervosa, his persistent depression, and his obsessive-compulsive disorder.

HOSPITAL COURSE: The patient continued to be relatively reluctant to cooperate in terms of his eating while on the Unit, and he began to secretly hide food even when he was under observation by staff members. He lost approximately four pounds during his first week in the hospital. Due to his continued weight loss, oppositional behavior, refusal to comply in relation to expectations of the Unit, and due to increasing fearfulness and concern about the patient's ability to sustain himself in the face of his self-deprivation, he will be transferred to the Medical Unit for further treatment in relation to his eating disorder. The patient was relatively passive initially about his transfer. He denied any sense of guilt or responsibility about being found with food in his pockets after meals, and he remained relatively negative and oppositional about any efforts to coerce him to eat or proceed with implementing a feeding tube in order to feed him. The patient remained angry at us for our unwillingness to allow him to starve to death. He became more negative toward the staff as it became clearer that we would not allow him to starve himself to death on Psychiatry. I discussed with him the various options in relation to feeding tubes versus eating. He continued to insist that he would not eat and would die of starvation.

His electrocardiogram on admission did indicate sinus brady-cardia with a rate of 46 beats per minute without other abnorma-lities. This bradycardia had been noted on previous admissions to the hospital and was not different in kind from the abnormalities noted previously.

Laboratory values indicated a mildly increased BUN of 36. SGOT was 375 with normal of 45, and this did appear to have increased during his stay in the hospital. Alkaline phosphatase was 178, which also appeared to have possibly increased mildly subsequent to his admission. As stated previously, there appeared to be some autolysis of his liver, and it was unclear to what extent this was related to his self-starvation. His other laboratory val-ues, which were abnormal, included decreased hematocrit at 32 on admission and 36 prior to transfer; this probably indicated overall an increasing degree of dehydration associated with his increase in self-starvation.

MEDICATIONS: The patient was on one can of Sustacal in the morning and 4 oz. at dinnertime. He was also on Prozac 20 mg p.o. b.i.d. and a multivitamin 1 b.i.d.

His vital signs remained relatively normal other than a hypo-thermia. The patient had previously been on blankets for his hypothermia, but he seemed to tolerate that more, presently, due to the chronicity of his hypothermia. There were no indications of any major complications associated with that, and it was unclear that there had been any damage to his kidneys or other organs as a result of that.

Overall, the patient seemed to show no improvement while in the hospital. In fact, he lost weight from his pre-admission level of 74 pounds down to 69 pounds. His condition overall was worsening, and he was physically stressed to the point that he needed to be on a Medical Unit in order to try to control the complications of his self-starvation. He will be transferred to Medicine for further care in relation to his self-starvation and in relation to his need for medical supervision for the complications of his anorexia nervosa. He will be transferred back to Psychiatry at such time as he is medically stable to continue active Ward Milieu therapy for his illness.

DISCHARGE DIAGNOSIS: 1. Anorexia nervosa.
2. Major depression.
3. Obsessive-compulsive disorder.
4. Uremia secondary to dehydration.
5. Bone marrow suppression.
6. Sinus bradycardia.
7. Anemia.
8. Increased liver function tests.

Stephen Wiener, MD
08/09/89; 08/25/89

NEWTON-WELLESLEY HOSPITAL
2014 Washington Street
Newton   Ma. 02162

NAME   KRASNOW, Michael

UNIT NO. 23 92 52

ADM.   6/28/89

DISCH.   8/9/89

DISCHARGE SUMMARY

This is a 20-year-old young man with a long history of severe anorexia nervosa. His mother, Gail Krasnow, is his guardian. He also has a history of an obsessive-compulsive disorder and depression. He was transferred from 3-Central because of weight loss, refusal to eat, hiding food, etc. He had recently been treated with Anafranil which is an experimental drug, for obsessive-compulsive disorder, however, not only was it not successful, but also resulted in increased LFT's. While on the medicine, he was followed by his psychiatrist, Dr. Wiener, as well as myself and he was intermittently followed by house staff. On 6/29, his weight was 68 1/2 pounds. The patient usually lay in bed and rarely got up and moved around. He was very regressed during the entire hospitalization. Tube feedings were commenced and the tube kept coming out. The patient said by accident, however, it was thought that the patient encouraged the tube to come out. However, the patient tried to bargain for a dietary program that did not involve tube feedings. The patient refused to drink extra fluids. His BUN went from 35 to 44 on 7/1. Feeding tube was replaced several times and removed several times. On 7/5, the patient had a respiratory arrest and a code was called. The patient was episodically apneic. He was peripherally treated with 02 and D-50 and became alert. He was transferred briefly to the ICU. Blood gases showed pH 7.45/37/161. In retrospect, it seems that the respiratory arrest was probably triggered by hypoglycemia. After stabilization, the patient was transferred back on 7/6 to medicine. The patient continued his behavior of pulling out the feeding tube; the feeding tube was put back and the patient was restrained. On 7/7, TPN was started and during this time, the patient was also noted to have undergone a spontaneous pneumo-thorax and also continued to have episodes of severe hypoglyce-mia with blood sugars in the 30s. On 7/8, the patient required insertion of a chest tube. On 7/8/89, the patient again had a code, was found to have an increased pneumothorax of 30 percent. The belief of the house staff at the time was that this was a respiratory arrest secondary to respiratory muscle failure with the pneumo-thorax. When I returned from my vacation on 7/10, I found his weight to be 73.9 and he was getting his I.V. TPN and had to be restrained with casts on both arms. He had a chest tube, and we are trying to get him into medical shape so that he could undergo ECT. The patient totally refused to eat or drink anything. On 7/12, his weight was 77 pounds and his crit was 21.0. He was getting an anemia workup plus he was getting blood transfusions for his severe anemia. He continued to be totally regressed and passive. On 7/14, his temperature rose to 100.0 and his chest tube drainage was cultured. His WBC count, however, had been only 1.1 and went to 1.5 with 58 percent polys. The patient was seen in consultation by Dr. O and was thought to have severe bone marrow failure as a result of his severe malnutrition. This was treated eventually with anabolic steroids and the patient made a good recovery with his bone marrow. By the 17th, although he was still critically ill, he refused to eat or drink at all. The patient's bone marrow during the crisis had shown a marked lack of cells. A surgical nutrition consult was obtained on 7/20 with the idea of putting in a feeding gastrostomy as we could not keep up the TPN forever. However, his temperature spiked on 7/22 to 101.0, 7/23 to 104.0, and it was felt that the patient had a line infection. He was treated with antibiotics for that. The antibiotic chosen was vancomycin. The advent of the line infection again redoubled our efforts to consider feeding gastrostomy, however, in light of the possibility of surgery, the patient was willing to bargain for some cooperation with his nutrition and agreed to eat some food. Dr. Wiener noted that the patient really felt that he gave in when he broke his record and started to eat again. He was very depressed over that. However, he did eat (although mini-mum amounts) and for a while, we were able to keep some of the tube feedings or at least I.V. fluids while he was eating, until he negotiated those away. He continued to have behavior which involved hiding food, such as hiding a pancake and also trying to pocket Sustacal cans. The patient was even upset about I.V. fluids replacement as he thought that that made him feel fat and, of course, he would not take anything PO midday as it made him feel fat. By 8/2, his LFT's were improved and his WBC count was improving. I added folate and B12 to his regimen after consultation with Dr. O. On 8/9, his weight was 69 3/4 pounds and he was cleared by anesthesia for ECT. It was decided that he should be transferred to psychiatry for ECT to have the extra milieu support, however on the 9th, he started to have some extra bowel movements and he complained of some abdominal pain, although he refused to take any Gelusil as it made him feel fat. He was indeed transferred to psychiatry and he continued to have hypoglycemic reactions. He was transferred to psychiatry either 8/9 or 8/10.

FINAL DIAGNOSIS: Severe anorexia nervosa, obsessive-compulsive personality disorder, severe malnutrition, bone marrow failure with anemia, respiratory arrest, spontaneous pneumothorax requiring chest tube drainage, severe episodes of hypoglycemia, line sepsis treated by vancomycin.

T. Spielberg, MD

BOURNEWOOD HOSPITAL
Name of Institution

Name KRASNOW, Michael A.   **No.** 44526

Date. ADM: 10/12/89
DIS: 10/23/89

DISCHARGE SUMMARY

The patient is a 20-year-old, white, single male with a history of severe anorexia nervosa and major depression with psychotic features including intense suicidality. The patient had previously been treated in Bournewood, both for his depression and for his eating disorder, [and] had most recently been here in July of 1988 where he had received ECT from Dr. N. The patient had subsequently remained out of the hospital and had a stable weight of 88 pounds until approximately March or April of 1989, when he again secretly started to lose weight and attempted to maintain this a secret by putting things in his pocket when he was being weighed, to offset his actual weight loss. He had been able to maintain a forty-hour/week job despite his weight loss until approximately June. At that time he was beginning to experience too many orthostatic problems from his weight loss and too much weakness from his loss of muscle mass. At that time he had been admitted to Newton-Wellesley Hospital, where he experienced numerous medical complications, being given an NG tube initially and subsequently a CVP line. He had a major respiratory problem when his lung was punctured from the CVP line, and he also had difficulties in terms of a systemic infection from that attempted feeding. He had very slowly regained weight and was at 74 pounds prior to his transfer to Bournewood on 10/12, almost four months after his initial admission. He continued to be negative about agreeing for treatment and to gain weight, but did agree to return to Bournewood due to the fact that he was no longer acutely medically ill and could not remain on the medical floor at Newton-Wellesley and could not contract adequately to be in their Eating Program there. His purpose for being transferred to Bournewood was to continue to maintain his safety from running away and starving himself to improve his motivation in accepting an eating disorder program, to continue to treat his major depression and his anorexia nervosa, and to establish additional weight gain to stabilize him medically. On admission he was on Navane 5 mg PO b.i.d., Prozac 40 mg PO b.i.d., and Benadryl 75 mg PO b.i.d. for symptoms associated with akathesia while on the Navane. Psychological goals were to have him deal with the persistent denial of the real risk of death by starvation if he continued to suppress his eating, and his needs to develop other ways to cope with stress and sense of loss in his relationship to [his] mother and the recent death of his father.

His admitting diagnoses were anorexia nervosa, severe malnutrition, recent pneumothorax, increased liver function tests, recent hypoglycemia, recent aplastic bone marrow, and major depression with psychotic features.

HOSPITAL COURSE: The patient initially presented in his usual negative way, felt restricted by being on the ITU, and felt that he was in a position to threaten to stage a new hunger strike if he was not immediately discharged. I discussed with him the lack of options other than his going to the eating program at McLeans, but he had apparently sabotaged that treatment plan by refusing to cooperate with the time frame that they had offered due to his resistance to agreeing to the caloric intake that they required for him to be accepted to the program. He continued to be relatively negative while he was in the hospital about gaining weight, continued to claim that his tray did not have adequate calories and this was the real explanation for his lack of weight gain, but he generally made no effort to increase his caloric intake beyond what was offered, even though there were multiple options for him to request additional food. He continued to remain in denial about his cachexia, self-starvation, and lack of compliance with expectations in relation to weight gain and improved health. He did continue to take his medications while he was in the hospital and showed some slight continuing improvement in his overall mood, probably related to his history of recent ECT at Newton-Wellesley by Dr. L. He continued to refuse groups at various times, especially when he was otherwise restricted to the unit for his failure to eat.

Medical complications did include a continuing persistent mild anemia, increased SGPT, which may have been associated with easy bruising due to his poor overall nutrition. His serum potassium did drop while he was in the hospital, and Dr. R put him on potassium supplements, which he generally refused to take. His EKG continued to manifest nonspecific ST-T changes although his atrial rate was slightly increased and there was no evidence of bradycardia while he was in the hospital. His lab tests other than the elevated SGPT were continuing to be normal with the exception of a low white count, but this was an increase over previously, and his bone marrow had been aplastic. He continued to show some evidence of mild liver toxicity, which may or may not have been related to his recent self-starvation. The patient continued to be relatively compliant about blood work and about talking with me, but was relatively negative in all other aspects.

His medications remained constant while he was in the hospital. He was on Navane 5 mg PO b.i.d., Prozac 40 mg PO b.i.d., Benadryl 75 mg PO b.i.d., multivitamin 1 PO q AM, and folic acid 1 mg PO q AM. He continued to refuse the supplement while he was in the hospital.

CONDITION ON DISCHARGE: Unimproved. He will be transferred back to Newton-Wellesley Hospital for further care and hopefully disposition to an eating disorder program. He will continue to be monitored closely in relation to his overall functioning at Newton-Wellesley, and hopefully for his acceptance to the Eating Disorder Program at Hahneman Hospital.

FINAL DIAGNOSIS: Anorexia Nervosa.
Major Depression with Psychotic Features.
Recent Bone Marrow Failure secondary to poor nutrition.
History of recent Sepsis with C-difficile infection.

Recent increased liver function tests related to malnutrition.
Severe Iron Deficiency Anemia.
Generalized Malnutrition.
Obsessive-Compulsive Disorder.

Stephen R. Wiener, MD
D: 11/09/89
T: 11/10/89

NEWTON-WELLESLEY HOSPITAL 2014 Washington Street Newton Ma. 02162	NAME KRASNOW, Michael
	UNIT NO.
	ADM.
DISCHARGE SUMMARY	DISCH. 10/12/89

This is a medical readmission for this patient transferred back to medicine from the psychiatric service on 8/11/89. This patient has had a long history of anorexia nervosa since the age of 14. His weight during most of this hospitalization ranged between 74 and 75 pounds. On the previous medical admission just before the psych admission, he had stopped eating completely for a month, requiring TPN. He had developed line sepsis because of that and had episodes of hypoglycemia and also had a pneumothorax. After being transferred back to the locked unit at NWH, he was too sick to stay on the psych floor and he could hardly walk or get around. He was obviously malnourished and he had had recent bone marrow failure because of the starvation, which miraculously improved, helped on by anabolic steroids. He had had a history of abnormal LFT's as a result of his malnutrition and Enafranil. He had repeated attacks of hypoglycemia believed to be secondary to the low glycogen stores with his malnutrition; however, it was a new diarrhea with elevated WBC count of 18,000, and the probable diagnosis of C-difficile, that precipitated his transfer back to the medical service. His Clostridia antibody test was positive and he was treated with Flagyl and Imodium successfully. Dr. N, a gastroenterologist, was consulted and agreed with the diagnosis and treatment. Because of the patient's severe depression and anhedonia and obsessive compulsive disorder with fixation on his calories and fixation on his body image, e.g., that he still felt fat even though he was grossly cachexic, it was the psychiatric plan of Dr. Wiener and Dr. L to try and get him ready for a course of ECT. Because of a severe iron deficiency anemia, he was treated with Inferon I.M. and had very good results with the correction of his

iron deficiency anemia. However, he still had episodes of hypoglycemia and at the time of transfer, he required I.V. fluids and glucose. The patient continued to need I.V. fluids and glucose because
of his tendency for hypoglycemia as a precaution because of his
cachetic state. He was given I.M. Decadron prior to ECT treatments, although it was later found that his serum cortisol tests
were normal and he did not have Addison's Disease. Before his
first ECT, the patient attempted to run away from the hospital and
he did walk away to the parking lot where he was apprehended
and brought back. He did write us a little note in which he apolo-
gized and which he did admit to lying when it came to food. His
serum cortisol levels were 60 and 24.2 which were consistent with
stress. He was continued on his ECT course getting the second one
on 8/18. He usually did very well with those except that he had a
little headache following the ECT. FBS was noted to be 47 and
therefore, he was given a trial on Diazoxide and small dose of
HCTZ to go with it. This was very successful and eliminated the
hypoglycemic episodes. The patient overall seemed to do better
with food with less confrontation and therefore, we attempted not
to supervise every little thing, but simply watched his weight every
other day. During his hospitalization, his weight was 71 pounds on
8/22 with 71 1/2 pounds at the time of discharge.

While in the hospital, because of his severe malnutrition and
elevated alkaline phosphatase, he was treated prophylactically
with Tums. A bone density study was WNL. The patient continued
to be extremely weak and was not appropriate even for suggestion
of transfer to the psych unit all during his ECT treatments. The
patient continued to eat around 1,200 calories a day but would not
eat more than that. He also would not eat mid-day, only morning
and evening meals. He continued being weak and dizzy during this
period. During his hospitalization, a discussion was had about a
paper that he had written some years ago on anorexia in which he
stressed his feelings of being out of control when he feels fat–he
feels inferior and out of control. When he is exercising willpower,
he feels superior and in control. It was my feeling that the total
control of any pleasure, resulting in his anhedonia, was a massive
defense against the obsessive-compulsive out of controlness. He

typically would not commit to anything, would not voice opinions on anything, would never admit to enjoying anything; his typical response would be a shrug. It was as if there was no "I" there. There was no individual; he appeared to be an observer in his own life. During his own hospitalization and the ECT treatments, he did seem to become a little more mellow, although he never relinquished his obsession with his eating disorder. He did become a little more friendly and less confrontational in general. As he began to eat a little more and as his weight came up a little bit, he no longer required the Dyazide and that was tapered and finally stopped. After his ECT was over, a consultation was made to see if either 3-Central or 3-East would take him back; however, they both refused as Michael refused to cooperate with their eating disorder programs. On 9/14, the patient reached his highest weight in the hospital of 77 1/2 pounds, however, he had been somewhat constipated and it was a question of whether or not that a real gain. By 9/19, his FBS was 79 off Dyazide and his albumin was still low at 2.9 showing the malnutrition. His potassium was 4.0. It was explained to the patient that in order to leave a hospital setting that he must be at a minimum of 80 pounds, however, the patient was totally unable to come even close to reaching that goal both psychologically or medically, and obviously still required psychiatric care as well as medical supervision because it was felt that the margin of safety was just not there under 80 pounds for him to be discharged out of a supervised hospital setting. The patient was also evaluated while in the hospital at McLean Hospital; however, the patient refused to cooperate with their program and would not agree to go there. During the hospital stay, the patient was able to go on passes to his mother's in late September and early October without any problems. Although he was not able to admit having any pleasure, his behavior indicated that he did look forward to those times and he even indicated that he wanted to get a birthday present for his brother, which was remarkable for him. By 9/27, it was noted that his anemia had been largely corrected; his hemoglobin was 12. He did go to the cemetery with his mother that day to see the grave of his father and he had "no feeling one way or the other," which is typical of Michael.

The patient was started on Navane by Dr. Wiener and that also appeared to be helpful in sort of mellowing him out. He was less confrontational, less angry, still obsessive about his food, and the calories that he was going to eat and would not change; however, on the Navane, he began to have (with a little Prozac) some problems with urinary retention and the Navane dose had to be decreased. In a few days before discharge, the patient reported that he had increased his calories to somewhere between 1400-1500 calories, however, this was not reflected in any change in his weight. His weight remained stable. He was re-evaluated again for treatment on 3-East and transfer; however, Ms. S, who evaluated him, was unable to obtain a commitment from Michael to cooperate with the eating disorders program and therefore, he could not be accepted there. Dr. Wiener then arranged for his transfer to Bournewood Hospital on 10/12/89 where he has agreed to continue his present caloric intake.

FINAL DIAGNOSIS:
1. Severe longstanding anorexia nervosa.
2. Probable psychotic core or outright psychosis.
3. Chronic depression and anhedonia.
4. Recent bone marrow failure secondary to malnutrition.
5. Recent series of hypoglycemia secondary to malnutrition.
6. History of recent sepsis and subsequent C-difficile infection treated.
7. Recent abnormal liver function tests that have returned to normal, believed to be the result of Enafranil and malnutrition.
8. Severe iron deficiency anemia treated.
9. Generalized malnutrition.

T. Spielberg, MD

NEWTON-WELLESLEY HOSPITAL
2014 Washington Street
Newton   Ma. 02162

NAME   KRASNOW, Michael

UNIT NO. 239252
               DOB: 4-27-69
ADM.   10-23-89

DISCHARGE SUMMARY

DISCH.   12-2-89

This is a readmission to NWH for this 20-year-old severe anorexic patient after having failed to cooperate with a program at Bournewood Hospital. He has had a history of severe hypoglycemia, anemia, bone marrow depression and elevated liver functions felt secondary to ethanol. His diagnoses included severe malnutrition secondary to the anorexia nervosa, depression, anemia, and hypoglycemia. While in the hospital he was followed by Dr. Wiener from Psychiatry, later on by Dr. M, from Psychology and myself.

On admission the patient's anemia was again documented, although it wasn't as severe as in the past. The sugar was 88. His hemoglobin was 10.2, went to 11.6. Liver function tests were within normal limits. We had the usual struggles over calories and the patient being very resistant to our advice. His weight at the time of admission was only 74 pounds. He was clearly in a state of malnutrition danger. In an effort to explore all alternatives for treatment, an application was also made for consideration for singulotomy at Massachusetts General Hospital. Patient was seen by Dr. K of Neurology to evaluate whether there were any neurological therapies as well as the singulotomy. It was recorded that the patient had had negative head CAT scans twice in the past.

While in the hospital the patient also refused to be considered for an eating disorder program at Hahneman and also refused another program at McLean Hospital. With daily input from Dr. Wiener, myself, and later on, beginning on 11-9-89 Dr. M, the patient gradually began to increase his calories and began to gain some weight. It was our attempt to do hypnotherapy with

Dr. M. However, Dr. M also became a therapist for the patient and the patient's mother as there seemed to be a pathological bond between the two of them. Dr. M also engaged in cognitive therapy as well. Although hypnotherapy was tried, the patient was not really able to concentrate enough to have that be effective. All during the hospitalization it was explained to Michael that the goal weight for discharge was 80 pounds. This was, of course, still cutting it close, but was something that I felt could be maintained and would give us a little margin for safety. Also, while in the hospital the patient was given high doses of Prozac (40 mg b.i.d.) as that has been shown in some recent studies to be effective for obsessive-compulsive disorder, which was part of his eating disorder psychopathology and he was receiving 40 mg b.i.d. He continued to refuse all "eating disorder programs." However, with our daily intervention he did manage to reach the 80-pound discharge weight on December 2, 1989 and was, therefore, discharged on that date.

His discharge medicines were Prozac 40 mg b.i.d., Benadryl 50 mg b.i.d., Slophy, folic acid, and multivitamins.

His postdischarge program involves seeing Dr. Wiener, Dr. M, and myself on a weekly basis.

FINAL DIAGNOSIS: Severe anorexia nervosa with severe malnutrition and obsessive-compulsive disorder, reactive depression, anemia, and history of hypoglycemia.

T. Spielberg, MD